Epilepsy
Patient & Family Guide

Third Edition

Epilepsy

Patient & Family Guide

Third Edition

Orrin Devinsky, MD

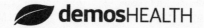

Library of Congress Cataloging-in-Publication Data

Epilepsy : patient and family guide / Orrin Devinsky. —3rd ed.
    p. cm.
Includes index.
ISBN-13: 978-1-932603-41-5 (pbk. : alk. paper)
ISBN-10: 1-932603-41-7 (pbk. : alk. paper)
    1. Epilepsy—Popular works. I. Devinsky, Orrin.
RC372.D48 2008
616.8'53—dc22

2007047858

Medicine is an ever-changing science undergoing continual development. Research and clinical experience are continually expanding our knowledge, in particular our knowledge of proper treatment and drug therapy. The authors, editors, and publisher have made every effort to ensure that all information in this book is in accordance with the state of knowledge at the time of production of the book.

Nevertheless, this does not imply or express any guarantee or responsibility on the part of the authors, editors, or publisher with respect to any dosage instructions and forms of application stated in the book. Every reader should examine carefully the package inserts accompanying each drug and check with a physician or specialist whether the dosage schedules mentioned therein or the contraindications stated by the manufacturer differ from the statements made in this book. Such examination is particularly important with drugs that are either rarely used or have been newly released on the market. Every dosage schedule or every form of application used is entirely at the reader's own risk and responsibility. The editors and publisher welcome any reader to report to the publisher any discrepancies or inaccuracies noticed.

. . . .

SPECIAL DISCOUNTS ON BULK QUANTITIES of Demos Medical Publishing books are available to corporations, professional associations, pharmaceutical companies, health care organizations, and other qualifying groups. For details, please contact:

Special Sales Department
Demos Medical Publishing
386 Park Avenue South, Suite 301
New York, NY 10016
Phone: 800-532-8663 or 212-683-0072
Fax: 212-683-0118
E-mail: orderdept@demosmedpub.com
. . . .

Printed in Canada
07 08 09 10   5 4 3 2 1

To my mom
For all your love and support

Contents

Foreword

The Epilepsy Foundation is pleased to welcome the third edition of *Epilepsy: Patient and Family Guide* as a valuable resource in empowering people with epilepsy, their caregivers and families. This book is an excellent source of accurate and insightful information on the medical aspects of epilepsy. It provides valuable information, which will enable you to work in collaboration with your neurologist and health care team toward the goal of no seizures and no side effects. This new edition also provides information on the exciting new developments in the treatment of epilepsy since the publication of the second edition in 2000, including expanded sections on alternative and dietary therapies, updates on mood disorders and vital information on sudden unexplained death syndrome.

Because epilepsy is not just a medical condition, but also something that impacts so many facets of daily life, this edition of *Epilepsy: Patient and Family Guide* covers topics such as employment, transportation, and legal issues – all areas of concern for adults with epilepsy. For parents and care givers, it also provides valuable information on the unique education issues for a child or young person with epilepsy and how parents can be effective advocates within the school system.

Readers will find the expanded information on mood disorders particularly valuable. Mood disorders among people with epilepsy, such as depression, are extremely common but often poorly diagnosed and under-treated. Studies suggest that one-third of people with hard to control seizures are clinically depressed and that depression is the biggest factor in quality of life, even more than seizure control. There is emerging evidence that mood disorders may have a common physiological basis with epilepsy. This is important as many people ascribe these feelings to the daily consequences of living with a chronic condition and fail to seek treatments that could be extremely effective.

The updated sections on alternative and dietary therapies are also quite important. While certain complementary therapies can help seizure control and improve quality of life, relying exclusively on non-medical therapies may have devastating, even life-threatening consequences. Dr. Devinsky has been at the forefront of exploring the use of complementary therapies for epilepsy and this new edition examines these therapies from a scientific standpoint and explains how to effectively utilize them.

While Epilepsy: Patient and Family Guide is both comprehensive and authoritative, no single book provides everything needed to win the battle against epilepsy. That's why it is important to work closely with your neurologist and health care team. If you are having seizures or problems with side-effects, ask questions – ask if there are other treatment options that might be better for you. Never settle and accept that "this is as good as it can get." If you have difficult to control seizures or side-effects, you may wish to see an "epileptolgist" — a neurologist who specializes in helping people with epilepsy.

Also remember that help is not limited to the physician's office. The Epilepsy Foundation provides many programs and services in your community to address the social, as well as medical aspects of epilepsy. For more information and to find the Epilepsy Foundation office that services your community, go to www.epilepsyfoundation.org.

The Epilepsy Foundation would like to recognize and thank Dr. Orrin Devinsky for making this excellent resource available to people and for donating the proceeds from this book to research. We believe that with an expanded commitment to research, a future with no seizures and no side-effects can be achieved. The Epilepsy Foundation will commit our very best so that one day there will be no more need for books – however excellent – on living with epilepsy.

ERIC R. HARGIS
President and Chief Executive Officer
Epilepsy Foundation

Preface

The goal of this book is to help people with epilepsy, as well as their families and friends, gain a better understanding about the disorder and how they can improve their quality of life. They are simple, achievable goals; yet they can be elusive. Information and understanding can facilitate those goals. A little information can be dangerous, but too little can be much more dangerous.

This book is organized so that it can be read from cover to cover or selected sections. Because epilepsy presents different problems and challenges at different stages of life, information pertaining to infants, children, adolescents, adults, women of childbearing age, and the elderly are treated separately. There is much to know about epilepsy—the nature and diversity of seizures, the psychological and social implications of seizures and the diagnosis of epilepsy, the educational and vocational impact of the disorder, and the medical, surgical, and alternative therapies. This third edition seeks to provide comprehensive, but focused information. As the internet becomes *the* source of information and endless detail, the need for accurate information on the internet is critical: epilepsy.com is an excellent source.

Knowledge is power. Yet information without context can be confusing and frightening. Perspective is essential. This book seeks to empower people with epilepsy with both information and perspective. For instance, anyone who reads the *Physician's Desk Reference,* which describes all prescription drugs, may be scared to learn about the extensive and potentially serious side effects of antiepileptic drugs. The risks, however, must be weighed against the benefits. For the vast majority of people, when a doctor recommends a drug, the positives far outweigh the negatives.

Persons with epilepsy should become advocates for themselves or their children who have epilepsy. Medical advice should make sense. Ask questions. If one is dissatisfied with the seizure control or side effects of therapy, they should discuss it with the doctor. The current regimen may truly be the best possible one, but sometimes a second opinion is helpful. Parents of a child with epilepsy must make sure the child's educational needs are met and the school district fulfills its legal obligations. Adults with epilepsy must make sure that the privilege to drive and their rights to employment are fairly considered.

I hope that this book helps to remove doubts and relieves fears that epilepsy can create, and builds confidence through knowledge. Finally, although most of my medical information about epilepsy comes from textbooks, journal articles, and professional lectures, the people I have cared for—my patients— have proved my greatest source of knowledge about living with epilepsy.

ORRIN DEVINSKY, MD

Acknowledgments

The information and thoughts that fill these pages are a collective effort, reflecting input from my colleagues' research, observations from the people I help care for, and my own views on epilepsy care. Several colleagues and friends have generously donated their time and helped ensure a more accurate and broader perspective. Many, many thanks to Jim Cloyd, Carol and Peter Camfield, Joyce Cramer, Jackie French, Eric Geller, Amy Koppelman, Ruben Kuzniecky, Warren Lammert, Kim Meador, Kim Parker, Kate Picco, Ley Sander, Blanca Vazquez, and Peter Widdeswalsh. Special thanks to George Lai, Kate Nearing, and Julie Devinsky who were invaluable in helping prepare the manuscript for publication. I would also like to thank Richard Johnson and the staff at Demos Medical Publishing who provided outstanding support throughout this project.

My deepest appreciation goes to my wife, Deborah and my daughters, Janna and Julie, for their endless inspiration and love.

I

Medical Aspects of Epilepsy

1 | An Overview of Epilepsy

E pilepsy has afflicted humans since the dawn of our species and was described in the earliest medical writings. Few medical conditions have attracted so much attention and generated so much controversy. Throughout history, people with epilepsy and their families have suffered unfairly because of the ignorance of others. Fortunately, the stigma of epilepsy has progressively declined in recent decades, and most people with epilepsy now lead normal lives.

The Greek physician Hippocrates wrote the first book on epilepsy, *On the Sacred Disease,* around 400 B.C. Hippocrates recognized that epilepsy was a brain disorder, and he refuted the ideas that seizures were a curse from the gods and that people with epilepsy held prophetic powers. False ideas die slowly—a 1494 handbook on witch-hunting, *Malleus Maleficarum,* written under papal authority, used seizures as a characteristic to identify witches. The *Malleus* fomented a wave of persecution and torture and the death of more than 200,000 women. In the early nineteenth century, asylums cared for people with epilepsy and psychiatric disorders, but the two groups were separated because seizures were considered contagious. In the early twentieth century, some U.S. states had laws forbidding people with epilepsy to marry or become parents, and some states permitted sterilization. We have come a long way.

Seizures and Epilepsy

A *seizure* is a brief, excessive discharge of brain electrical activity that changes how a person feels, senses, thinks, or behaves. During an epileptic seizure, the regulatory systems that maintain the normal balance between stimulation (excitation) and dampening (inhibition) of nerve cell activity break down. For example, there may be a loss of inhibitory activity or an overproduction of an excitatory neurotransmitter that cause a group of abnormal cells to fire excessively. These in turn may stimulate neighboring cells or cells with which they have strong connections. Ultimately, large populations are abnormally activated all at once (synchronously). That is, the electrical discharges of many cells become linked, creating a storm of activity.

Seizures cause an incredible range of effects, including (1) sensation of "pins and needles" in the thumb for 20 seconds, (2) hallucinations of smelling burned rubber and hearing a buzz with a rising abdominal sensation followed by staring with loss of awareness for several minutes, and (3) loss of consciousness with a fall and convulsive movements. Many patients consider only their tonic-clonic (grand mal) convulsive seizures to be "seizures" and regard other seizures such as jerks and auras to be "warnings or minor spells." However, if abnormal brain electrical discharges change behavior, no matter how subtly, they are seizures.

Epilepsy is a disorder in which a person has two or more seizures without a clear cause, such as alcohol withdrawal. In other words, epilepsy is a condition of *recurrent* and *unprovoked seizures*. The seizures may result from a hereditary tendency or a brain injury. The cause is often unknown, particularly in otherwise healthy people without apparent risk factors.

For many persons, the term "epilepsy" is more serious and frightening than "seizure disorder." However, epilepsy is a seizure disorder. Accepting the condition for what it is, name and all, is often the first step toward leading a normal life. Epilepsy refers to all individuals with two or more seizures, regardless of seizure severity, the age at which the seizures began, or their origin, except for clearly identified causes such as heart problems, alcohol withdrawal, extremely low blood sugar, or drug use. For example, some patients with abnormal heart rhythms may have a lack of blood flow due to their heart problem. This can result in loss of consciousness and a convulsive episode that looks exactly like a tonic-clonic seizure, but it is not an epileptic seizure. In other cases, a woman with diabetes may take took much insulin on two occasions and suffer seizures, but she has hypoglycemic seizures, not epilepsy. These are *provocative causes* – if you remove the provocation, you eliminate the chance of a seizure. In contrast, a man with a head injury who has two seizures after a *provocative factor* such as sleep deprivation has epilepsy.

Some Common Questions and Misunderstandings About Epilepsy

I had one seizure, will I get epilepsy?

After a single seizure, the chances of another are about 50%. People with a known brain injury and those with abnormalities on their neurologic examination, magnetic resonance imaging (MRI), computed tomography (CT) scan, or electroencephalogram (EEG) are more likely to have another seizure, whereas those with normal findings are much less likely to have a second seizure.

Do not fear the word epilepsy!

People see you through your eyes. If you are afraid of epilepsy, they will be afraid of it. It is a neurologic disorder; if you are comfortable in talking about it, then almost everyone else will be. There will be exceptions, but those individuals are unlikely to be more sympathetic to someone with a "seizure disorder" than "epilepsy."

Epilepsy and seizures are common

More than 2 million Americans have epilepsy; 9 million will have epilepsy at some time in their life. One in 11 people will have at least one seizure during their lifetime. Epilepsy afflicts all age groups, with the highest rates of new cases occurring during childhood and after age 60 years. It is slightly more common in males.

What causes epilepsy?

Anything that injures nerve cells in the brain can cause epilepsy. But in many cases we don't know the cause. Some patients have brain injuries from head trauma, infection, or other causes, such as an abnormal brain architecture found on MRI. In some people, genetic factors are likely responsible, but paradoxically, in most of these, there is no one else in the immediate family with epilepsy.

Most people with epilepsy enjoy full seizure control and lead normal lives

Most people with epilepsy have normal intelligence, behavior, and enjoy seizure freedom with few medication side effects. Approximately 70% of children with epilepsy will outgrow it. Overall, for children and adults with recently diagnosed epilepsy or those whose seizures are controlled with medication, the outlook is very positive.

In 30% of patients, seizures are not fully controlled

This "refractory" or medically resistant group is a diverse population. Some people have infrequent seizures such as occasional jerks affecting their shoulders or arms (myoclonic seizures) or dreamy feelings (simple partial seizures) that do not interfere with their lives. Other patients have only rare tonic-clonic seizures in sleep. Yet many people suffer from disabling seizures and often medication side effects despite the best efforts of their doctors and trials of many medications.

The consequences of epilepsy extend beyond seizures

Many patients and doctors equate the disorder—epilepsy—with the symptoms—seizures. However, epilepsy causes problems affecting other parts of a person's life. These effects vary with the severity of epilepsy. If seizures are controlled with low doses of medication, there should be few effects. However, even well-controlled patients may still fear the uncertainty and loss of control over when a seizure might happen. Medication side effects are often a problem. For those with poorly controlled seizures, restrictions on driving or operating dangerous machinery, injuries from a fall, stigma, and other issues adversely affect quality of life. Quality-of-life issues are particularly relevant in epilepsy, the paradigm of a chronic disorder in which the symptoms (seizures) are infrequent while effects of medication and psychosocial problems are continuous and pervasive.

Is there anything wrong with the word epileptic?

The word "epileptic" should not be used to describe someone who has epilepsy, as it defines a person by one trait. Labels are powerful and create limits and negative stereotypes. It is better to refer to someone as "a person with epilepsy" or to a group of people as "people with epilepsy." It is fine, however, to say someone has had an epileptic seizure.

Does epilepsy cause progressive deterioration of mental and behavioral function?

No! Most people with epilepsy have normal intelligence and behavioral function. There are some people with epilepsy, however, who have associated with brain injuries that cause neurologic impairments, including cognitive problems. For patients with poorly controlled epilepsy, especially those with recurrent tonic-clonic seizures over many years, the seizures can contribute to memory impairment and psychiatric problems.

Does epilepsy cause mental illness?

Although most people with epilepsy enjoy normal mental health, there is a higher rate of behavioral problems such as depression and anxiety among individuals with epilepsy. The relationship is complex. Patients with depression are more likely to develop seizures and epilepsy, and those with epilepsy are more likely to develop depression than the general population. For patients with epilepsy, depression and other behavioral problems are more common among those with poorly controlled seizures.

Do seizures damage the brain?

Single brief seizures do not cause brain damage. Although tonic-clonic (grand mal) seizures lasting longer than 20 minutes may injure the brain, there is no evidence that short seizures cause permanent injury to the brain. Rarely, prolonged or repetitive complex partial seizures may cause brain injury.

Memory problems and other intellectual problems can occur after a seizure. These problems result from temporary impairment of brain function. In some people there may be a cumulative, negative effect of many seizures, especially tonic-clonic seizures, on brain function.

If I have epilepsy, will my child have it?

The vast majority of cases are not inherited, although some types are genetically transmitted. Most of these types are easily controlled with medication.

Is epilepsy a lifelong problem?

Most people with epilepsy require medication for only a small portion of their lives. For many forms of epilepsy in children and adults, when the person has been free of seizures for 2–4 years, medications can often be slowly withdrawn and discontinued under a doctor's supervision.

Does epilepsy affect the life span?

People with infrequent seizures have death rates comparable to the general population, and the average person with epilepsy has a normal life span. However, epilepsy is associated with a slight reduction in life expectancy, partly due to conditions such as stroke and brain tumors. The increased risk of death is mainly limited to the first decade after diagnosis.

Epilepsy should not be a barrier to success

Epilepsy is perfectly compatible with a normal, happy, and full life. The person's quality of life, however, may be affected by the frequency and severity of the seizures, medications, and associated disorders. Some types of epilepsy are harder to control than others. Living successfully with epilepsy requires a positive outlook, a supportive environment, and good medical care. Coping with the reaction of other people to the disorder can be the most difficult part of living with epilepsy.

How do I balance protecting my child with fostering independence?

Children with epilepsy should be treated like other children, with some precautions governed by the frequency and severity of seizures. Acquiring a positive outlook may be easier said than done, especially for those who have grown up with insecurity and fear. Perhaps the greatest gift a parent can give a child is self esteem. Many children with chronic medical illnesses have low self-esteem, due partly to the reactions of others and to parental concern that fosters dependence and insecurity.

2 | Classification and Features of Epileptic Seizures

Classification of Seizures

Epileptic seizures can be broadly divided into two groups: (1) primary generalized and (2) partial (Table 2.1). Primary generalized seizures begin with a widespread, excessive electrical discharge simultaneously involving both sides of the brain. In contrast, partial seizures begin with an abnormal electrical discharge restricted to one, or several, discrete area(s). Distinguishing primary generalized seizures from partial seizures is critical because the diagnostic tests and the drugs used to treat these disorders differ. A description of what happened before, during, and after the seizure, as well as recordings of electrical activity generated by the brain (*brain waves*), helps to determine the type of seizure. In particular, the first few seconds of a seizure provide important clues. Brain waves are recorded on the EEG. It can detect abnormal electrical impulses in people with epilepsy (see Chapter 9). In primary generalized seizures, the EEG shows a widespread increase in electrical activity. In partial seizures, the brain waves show a more restricted, or local, increase of electrical activity. However, the EEG may be normal in people with epilepsy, and occasionally it shows epilepsy waves in people who have never had a seizure.

Hereditary factors are more important in primary generalized seizures than in partial seizures. In some cases, it can be difficult to distinguish

Table 2.1. Classification of Epileptic Seizures
Primary Generalized Seizures
Absence seizures
Typical
Atypical
Myoclonic seizures
Atonic seizures
Clonic seizures
Tonic seizures
Tonic-clonic seizures
Partial Seizures (Seizures Originating in Specific Parts of the Brain)
Simple partial seizures (consciousness not impaired)
With motor symptoms (jerking, stiffening)
With somatosensory (touch) or specialized sensory (smell, hearing, taste, sight) symptoms
With autonomic symptoms (heart rate change, internal sensations)
With psychic symptoms (déja vu, dreamy state)
Complex partial seizures (consciousness impaired, automatisms usually present)
Beginning as simple partial seizures
Beginning with impairment of consciousness
Partial seizures secondarily generalized to tonic-clonic seizures

primary generalized seizures from partial seizures, as many of their features overlap. For example, a tonic-clonic seizure may begin as a primary generalized seizure or as a partial seizure, and a staring spell can be an absence seizure (a type of primary generalized seizure) or a complex partial seizure (see below).

Level of Consciousness During Seizures

Determining whether the consciousness is preserved, impaired, or lost during a seizure helps classify the seizure type and allows recommendations about what activities are safe to pursue. Neurologically speaking, consciousness is the ability to respond and to remember. People with some kinds of seizures do not recall the seizure and don't even know that they have had a seizure. Others are aware that they had a seizure, but are convinced that they had no loss or impairment of consciousness when, in fact, they did. Therefore, it is helpful to have a family member or friend test the person during a seizure by asking him or her to follow commands such as "show me your left hand" and "remember the word yellow." If the person can follow the command and remember the word, consciousness is preserved, at least during the time tested.

Although neurologists describe consciousness during seizures as either impaired or preserved, the borderline between these categories is blurred. The degree of impairment or preservation of consciousness may vary between seizures. A patient may report being "half conscious, present but absorbed in my interior thoughts". Consciousness may be affected if either responsiveness or memory is impaired during an attack, but these two criteria do not have the same importance for the person's functioning. For example, during a seizure someone may be able to respond well but later be unable to recall some details of the seizure. In such cases, the person may be able to operate dangerous equipment safely or perform complex tasks during a seizure. Some seizures, however, may impair a person's ability to move voluntarily. The person is unable to speak or raise his or her hand when asked but may be able to recall the entire event. In this example, consciousness is preserved and motor control is impaired.

Primary Generalized Seizures

Primary generalized seizures simultaneously begin from both sides of the brain. The principal types are absence seizures, atypical absence seizures, myoclonic seizures, atonic seizures, clonic seizures, tonic seizures, and tonic-clonic seizures.

Absence Seizures

> Frank, a 7-year-old boy, often "blanks out" for a few seconds, and sometimes for 10–20 seconds. His teacher calls his name, but he doesn't seem to hear her. He usually blinks repetitively, and his eyes may roll up a bit, but with the short seizures he just stares. Then he is right back where he left off. Some days he has more than 50 spells.

Absence (petit mal) seizures are brief episodes of staring with impairment of awareness and responsiveness. The episode usually lasts less than 10 seconds, but can last as long as 20 seconds and, rarely, longer. The seizure begins and ends suddenly. There is no warning before the seizure, and immediately afterward the person is alert and attentive and often unaware that a seizure has occurred. These spells commonly begin in children between 4 and 14 years of age. In approximately 75% of these children, absence seizures do not continue after age 18. Absence seizures can often be provoked by rapid breathing (hyperventilation), and they usually can be reproduced in the doctor's office with this technique if the patient is not taking medication. However, absence seizures are uncommon with rapid breathing during exercise. Children with absence seizures have normal development and intelligence but may have higher rates of behavioral, educational, and social problems than other children.

Simple absence seizures are just "stares." During complex absence seizures, staring is accompanied by some change in muscle activity such as eye blinks, slight tasting movements of the mouth, or rubbing the fingers together. Complex absence seizures are more common with if the seizure lasts more than 10 seconds.

The EEG is extremely helpful in diagnosing absence seizures. In most cases, a characteristic generalized spike-and-wave discharge at three to four per second is found, especially during hyperventilation (see Chapter 9, Fig. 13). Neuroimaging tests such as CT and MRI (see Chapter 9) are normal in children with absence seizures, so they are usually not needed. Absence seizures may be confused with complex partial seizures (discussed later). Absence seizures are usually briefer (less than 20 seconds) and are not associated with a warning (aura) or postepisode symptoms such as tiredness.

Atypical Absence Seizures

> It is hard for me to tell when Kathy is having one of her staring spells. During the spells, she doesn't respond as quickly as at other times. The problem is that she often doesn't respond so quickly, and she often just stares when she is not having an absence seizure.

The staring spells of *atypical absence seizures* also occur predominantly in children, and usually begin before 6 years of age. In contrast with typical absence seizures, atypical absence seizures often begin and end gradually (over seconds), often last more than 10 seconds (the usual duration is 5–30 seconds), and usually are not provoked by rapid breathing. The child stares but often has only a partial reduction in responsiveness. Eye blinking or slight jerking movements of the lips may occur. Affected children often have lower than average intelligence and other seizures types (myoclonic, tonic, and tonic-clonic types). Atypical absence seizures can be hard to distinguish from the child's usual behavior, especially in those with lower intelligence.

Most children with these seizures have an abnormal EEG, with slow spike-and-wave discharges even when they are not having a seizure. Atypical absence seizures often continue into later childhood.

Myoclonic Seizures

> In the morning I get these "jumps." My arms just go flying up for a second. I may spill my coffee or drop a book. Occasionally my mouth shuts for a split second. Sometimes I get a few of these jumps in a row. Once I have been up for a few hours I never get any more of these jumps.

Myoclonic seizures are brief, shock-like jerks of a muscle or group of muscles. Myoclonus may occur in people who do not have epilepsy. For example, as many people fall asleep, their body suddenly jerks. These are *sleep jerks* or *benign nocturnal myoclonus*. Abnormal forms of myoclonus include epileptic or nonepileptic types.

Epileptic myoclonus usually causes abnormal movements on both sides of the body at the same time. The neck, shoulders, upper arms, body, and upper legs are usually involved. Some patients describe a "shiver." Myoclonic seizures occur in a variety of disorders that have different sets of characteristics. How well these seizures can be controlled depends on which of these disorders (syndromes) affects the individual (see Chapter 3).

Myoclonic seizures in the juvenile myoclonic epilepsy syndrome most often involve the neck, shoulders, and upper arms. The seizures often occur within 1 hour after awakening. They may be provoked by flashing lights, or less commonly by reading or other specific tasks. They are usually well controlled with medication, but the disorder is often lifelong.

The Lennox-Gastaut syndrome often includes myoclonic, tonic, and other seizure types that can be difficult to control (see Chapter 3). These myoclonic seizures may cause the person to fall.

Atonic Seizures

> Bob's "drop" seizures are his biggest problem. He falls to the ground and often hits his head and bruises his body. Even if I'm right next to him and prepared, I may not catch him. The helmet is great, but he often forgets to put it on before he gets out of bed.

In an *atonic seizure*, the person suddenly loses muscle strength. The eyelids may droop, the head may nod, objects may be dropped, or the person may fall to the ground. Atonic seizures usually begin in childhood. Although they last less than 15 seconds, they frequently cause sudden falls, so injury is common. When patients with "drop seizures" are studied carefully, however, many actually have *tonic* seizures (associated with muscle contraction; see below), not *atonic* seizures.

Clonic Seizures

Clonic seizures are rare and consist of rhythmic jerking movements of the arms and legs. These may be generalized, convulsive seizures with jerking (clonic) movements on both sides of the body but without the stiffening (tonic) component seen in the more common tonic-clonic seizures. Clonic seizures are not followed by a prolonged period of confusion or tiredness. Some tonic-clonic seizures are preceded by jerking movements (clonic-tonic-clonic seizures) in juvenile myoclonic epilepsy.

Tonic Seizures

> Jeff just stiffens up. Both arms are raised over his head, and he grimaces, as if someone is pulling on his cheeks. The episodes last less than a minute, but if he is standing he may lose his balance and fall. These seizures don't knock him out like the grand mals, but if he has a few close together, he is often tired.

Tonic seizures, usually lasting less than 20 seconds, are associated with sudden stiffening movements of the body, arms, or legs, and involve both sides of the body. They are more common during sleep or in the transition into or out of sleep. The person often will fall if the seizure occurs while she is standing. Tonic seizures are most common in children who have lower than average intelligence, but can occur in any child or adult.

Tonic-Clonic Seizures

> These seizures frighten me. They last only a minute or so, but it feels like an eternity. I can often tell they are coming because she is more cranky and out of sorts. Heather shrieks with this unnatural cry, falls, and every muscle in her body tenses. Her teeth clench. I know she can't, but I still worry she will swallow her tongue. She is pale and, later, a slight bluish color. Shortly after she falls, her arms and upper body start to jerk. This is the longest part. Then it finally stops and she is out cold.

Tonic-clonic (grand mal) seizures are convulsive seizures. The person briefly stiffens (tonic phase) and loses consciousness, falls, and often utters a cry. It is not a cry from pain, but from air being forced through the contracting vocal cords. This is followed by jerking (clonic phase) of the arms and legs. The seizures usually last 1–3 minutes. There may be excessive saliva production, sometimes described as "foaming" at the mouth. Biting of the tongue or cheek may cause bleeding. Loss of urine or, rarely, a bowel movement may occur. Afterward the person is tired and confused for a period of minutes to hours and often goes to sleep, but he or she may be agitated or depressed. The time immediately after the seizure is called the *postictal* period. First aid is discussed in Chapter 10.

Tonic-clonic seizures lasting more than 5 minutes or recurring in a series of three or more seizures without the person returning to a normal state in between is a dangerous condition called *convulsive status epilepticus*. This condition requires medical treatment, such as rectal diazepam or buccal midazolam, or medical help should be obtained (see Chapter 10). The exact duration of continuous seizure activity that is harmful to the brain is not well defined; children appear to tolerate seizures lasting longer than 5 minutes better than adults do.

Partial Seizures

Partial seizures begin with an abnormal burst of electrical activity in a restricted area of the brain. Most partial seizures arise from the temporal or frontal lobes. Head injury, brain infections, stroke, and brain tumors are common causes. In some cases, hereditary factors are also important. In many cases, no cause can be identified.

Partial seizures are divided into two main types, depending on whether consciousness is fully preserved. During *simple partial seizures*, the person is alert, is able to respond to questions or commands, and can remember what occurs. During *complex partial seizures*, the ability to pay attention or to respond to questions or commands is impaired to some degree. Often there is no memory of what happened during all or part of the seizure. The distinction between simple and complex partial seizures is critical, because the ability to drive, operate dangerous equipment, swim alone, and perform other activities usually has to be restricted in people with uncontrolled complex partial seizures. A third type of partial seizure is one that spreads widely to become a secondarily generalized tonic-clonic (grand mal) seizure.

Simple Partial Seizures

> I almost enjoy them. The feeling of déjà vu, like I have lived through this moment, and I even know what is going to be said next. Everything seems brighter and more alive.

> It is a pressure that begins in my stomach and rises up to my chest and I smell the same odor, something burnt, definitely unpleasant. At the same time I feel nervous.

Simple partial seizures can cause a remarkably diverse group of symptoms. In some cases, the symptoms are not recognized as a seizure, because they can also be caused by other factors. For example, abdominal discomfort is usually from a gastrointestinal disorder, but it also can be a symptom of a partial seizure. Tingling in the little finger that spreads to the forearm may come from a seizure, a migraine, or a peripheral nerve disorder (e.g., "pinched nerve").

Motor seizures affect muscle activity. Most often, the body stiffens, or the muscles begin to jerk in one area of the body such as a finger or the wrist. The abnormal movements may remain restricted to one body part or may spread to involve other muscles on the same side or both sides of the body. Some partial motor seizures cause weakness; this can affect the vocal apparatus and impair speech. Motor seizures may also include coordinated actions such as laughter or automatic hand movements.

Sensory seizures cause changes in sensation. Most often, a person has a hallucination, the sensation of something that is not there, such as a feeling of "pins and needles" in a finger, tasting "bitter," or seeing a colored pinwheel. The abnormal sensations may remain restricted to one area or may spread. There also may be an illusion, the distortion of a true sensation. For example, a parked car appears to be moving, or a person's voice is muffled. Hallucinations and illusions can involve all types of sensations, including touch (numbness, pins and needles), smell (often an unpleasant odor), taste, vision (a spot of light, a scene with people), hearing (a click or ringing, a person's voice), and orientation in space (a floating or spinning feeling).

Autonomic seizures change automatically controlled bodily functions such as heart rate or sweating. The emotion (limbic) system is closely connected to the autonomic nervous system. This is why strong emotions such as fear are associated with increases in the heart rate and breathing rate, sweating, and a sinking feeling in the chest. It is also the basis of why we say such things as "In my heart, it's right," or "I have a gut feeling." Partial seizures commonly arise from the limbic areas. Therefore, autonomic changes are common during partial seizures. Autonomic partial seizures can cause a strange or unpleasant sensation in the abdomen, chest, or head; changes in heart rate or breathing rate; sweating; or goose bumps.

Psychic seizures affect how we think, feel, and experience things. These seizures can impair language function, causing garbled speech, inability to find the right word, or difficulty understanding spoken or written language, as well as problems with time perception and memory. Psychic seizure can cause sudden and often intense emotions such as fear, anxiety, depression, or happiness. Unlike normal emotional feelings that are triggered by an environmental event or internal thought, psychic seizures provoke spontaneous emotions that "come out of the blue." Other psychic seizures can make a person feel as if: they experienced or lived through this moment before (*déja vu*), familiar things are strange and foreign (*jamais vu*), one is not oneself (depersonalization), the world is not real (derealization), or one is in a dream or watching oneself from outside one's body.

Complex Partial Seizures

> Harold's spells begin with a warning; he says he is going to have a seizure and usually sits down. I ask him what he feels, but he either doesn't answer or just says, "I feel it." Then he makes a funny face, with "surprise" and "distress." He just stares. I call his name, and he may look at me when I call, but he never answers. During this part, he may make these "tasting" mouth movements. He often grabs the arm of the chair and squeezes it. Other times, he touches his shirt, as if he is picking lint off, even though it's clean. It lasts a minute, and as he comes back he keeps asking questions. He never remembers what he asks or says right after the seizure. He is tired afterward; if he has two in the same day he goes to sleep after the second one.

> Susan's seizures usually occur during sleep. She makes this grunting sound, like she is clearing her throat. She sits up in bed, opens her eyes, and stares. She sometimes clasps her hands together. I ask her what she is doing, but she doesn't say a word. Within a minute, she lies back down and goes back to sleep.

With *complex partial seizures (psychomotor or temporal lobe seizures)*, consciousness is impaired but not lost. The person typically stares but cannot respond to questions or commands, or responds incompletely and inaccurately. Automatic movements (*automatisms*) occur in many complex partial seizures. Automatisms can involve the mouth and face (lip smacking, chewing, tasting, and swallowing movements), the hands and arms (fumbling, picking, tapping, or clasping movements), vocalizations (grunts, repetition of words or phrases), or more complex acts (walking or mixing foods in a bowl). Other, less common automatisms include laughing,* screaming, crying, running, shouting, bizarre and sometimes sexual-appearing movements, and disrobing. Complex partial seizures usually last from 20 seconds to 2 minutes. Auras (simple partial seizures) are common and typically occur seconds before consciousness is altered. After the seizure, lethargy and confusion are common, but usually last less than 15 minutes. Complex partial seizures occur in persons of all ages.

Some people are unaware that they have had a complex partial seizure. Many of the symptoms are so subtle that others may just think the person is "thinking about something," "daydreaming," or "spacing out." These episodes can cause memory lapses, and someone may perform complex activities but have no recall of them. One doctor found himself in a hospital lobby and realized that he was supposed to examine a patient. He went to see the patient and examined her. To his amazement, when he went to write his note, he found that he had just been there and correctly diagnosed pneumonia, but had no recollection of ever having seen the patient. He probably examined her and made his notes just before a complex partial seizure, which "wiped out" his memory for a short period.

---

* Seizures with laughing automatisms are referred to as *gelastic seizures*. They can occur with partial seizures arising from temporal or frontal lobes or from lesions such as a benign tumor affecting the hypothalamus. Patients with hypothalamic lesions and gelastic seizures may experience puberty at an early age and exhibit aggressive behavior.

In the wrong setting, automatic behaviors with impaired consciousness could be dangerous: a person could walk into the street without awareness of the cars. This is very rare.

Some unusual automatisms cause embarrassment and problems. For some persons, these automatisms are typical during their seizures. Others only rarely have embarrassing behavior such as disrobing at work. This was a problem, for example, in a person I cared for who worked in an elementary school. As with most other aspects of epilepsy, special precautions can be taken to help minimize the negative effects of such behaviors.

Secondarily Generalized Seizures

They start with a tingling in the right thumb. Then the thumb starts jerking. In a few seconds, the whole right hand is jerking, and I learned to start rubbing and scratching my forearm. Sometimes I can stop the seizure this way. Other times the jerking spreads up the arm. When it reaches the shoulder, I pass out and people tell me that my whole body shakes.

I see this colored ball on my right side. The ball seems to grow and fill up my whole view. As the ball grows, everything becomes like a dream, and I don't feel real. It is the strangest feeling. The seizure can just stop, and my vision is just a little blurry, or it can go all the way, fall to the floor and have a grand mal.

When the seizure discharge starts in a localized area but later spreads to involve both sides of the brain, the partial seizure may become a *secondarily generalized tonic-clonic seizure*. Secondarily generalized seizures are common, occurring in more than 30% of children and adults with partial epilepsy. Patients may or may not recall an aura, and witnesses may first observe a complex partial seizure that progresses to a tonic-clonic seizure. A secondarily generalized tonic-clonic seizure may be difficult to distinguish from a primary generalized tonic-clonic seizure, especially if it is not witnessed or occurs during sleep. (Most convulsive seizures in sleep begin as partial seizures.) The EEG and MRI can help distinguish these seizure types.

The Postictal Period

The period immediately after a seizure, the postictal period, varies depending on the type, duration, and intensity of the seizure, as well as other factors. Postictal symptoms can help distinguishdifferent types of seizures in which staring is a major component. Absence seizures are not followed by any postictal symptoms—when the seizure ends, activity resumes as if nothing had happened. After most complex partial seizures, the person is slightly confused and tired, usually for less than 5–15 minutes. Immediately after a tonic-clonic seizure, the person appears limp and unresponsive, and may be pale or bluish (cyanotic). On awakening, the person often complains of muscle soreness and headache and of pain in the tongue or cheek if those areas were bitten. The person may be confused and tired. Often those who have had a tonic-clonic seizure awaken briefly and then go to sleep.

Other symptoms follow some seizures. Weakness of an arm or leg after a partial motor or tonic-clonic seizure may be Todd's paralysis. Seizures may also be followed by impairments in vision, touch sensation, language, and other functions. Often the nature of the postictal problem can help identify the area where the seizure began. For example, weakness in the right arm and leg may follow a seizure that began in, or near, the motor area of the left hemisphere. These postictal symptoms often improve after minutes to hours, but can be more prolonged.

For some patients, postictal symptoms such as fatigue, depression, confusion, memory impairment, or headache can be more troublesome than the seizure itself. In such cases, changes in antiepileptic drugs may not alter the seizures but may minimize the postictal symptoms. In other cases, treatment of specific symptoms such as postictal headache (using medications for migraine headache, for example) can be helpful.

Change in Seizure Patterns

Many people have more than one type of seizure. For example, one person may have both simple and complex partial seizures, or absence, myoclonic seizures and tonic-clonic seizures. In addition, the features of each type of seizure may change from seizure to seizure. More often, the features change over months or years. For instance, a person's simple partial seizures that precede tonic-clonic seizures may change from an unpleasant smell and a strange stomach sensation to simply a sensation of chest discomfort, or there may no longer be any warning.

Changes in a person's seizures may result from changes in the patterns of spread of the abnormal electrical discharge. In the case of the person whose aura (simple partial seizure) no longer precedes the tonic-clonic seizure, the area from which the seizure begins and the intensity of the discharge probably have not changed, but the electrical activity may have taken other pathways that allow it to spread more rapidly. In this case, the absence of a warning may prevent the person from avoiding injury even though the seizure is no more severe than before.

Those who have had mild seizures, such as simple partial or absence seizures, later may experience tonic-clonic seizures. In some instances, the change in seizure type may result from factors such as missed medication or lack of sleep. For others, it is just the way their disorder develops; they have always had a small chance of having a tonic-clonic seizure.

We don't know exactly why seizure patterns change over time. There may be some changes in the brain such as reorganization of connections or an increase or decrease in the concentrations of certain chemicals. If seizures become more frequent or more severe, a neurologic checkup is advisable.

3 | Classification of Epileptic Syndromes

E pileptic syndromes are defined by a cluster of features, including seizure type(s), age when seizures begin, EEG findings, and prognosis (outlook). Classifying an epileptic syndrome can provide information on how long seizures will persist and what medications will help or hurt. Common epileptic syndromes include febrile seizures, benign rolandic epilepsy, juvenile myoclonic epilepsy, infantile spasms, Lennox-Gastaut, reflex epilepsies, temporal lobe epilepsy, and frontal lobe epilepsy. Rare syndromes include generalized epilepsy-febrile seizures plus, progressive myoclonic epilepsies, mitochondrial disorders, Landau-Kleffner syndrome, and Rasmussen's syndrome.

Febrile Seizures

Tommy was just 14 months old. He caught a bad cold from a child in his playgroup. He had a fever and runny nose. He was taking a nap when I heard this strange banging sound. I ran into his room, and his whole body was stiff and shaking. Those 5 minutes were the longest 5 minutes of my life. He has never had another one, and doesn't need any seizure medication. Now when he has a fever I give him Tylenol. ·

Children aged 3 months to 6 years may have tonic-clonic seizures when they have a high fever. These febrile seizures occur in 2–5% of children. In some families there is a hereditary tendency toward febrile seizures. The usual situation is a healthy child with normal development, aged 6 months to 2 years, who has a viral illness with high fever. As the child's temperature rapidly rises, he or she has a generalized tonic-clonic seizure. In contrast with tonic-clonic seizures in later childhood and adulthood, febrile seizures often last longer than 5 minutes. In most instances, hospitalization is not necessary, although a prompt medical consultation is essential after the first seizure.

The prognosis for febrile seizures is excellent. There is no reason for a child who has had a single febrile seizure to receive antiepileptic drugs unless the seizure was unusually long or other problems are identified. Recurrence rates (chances of another seizure) vary from 50% if the seizure occurred before age 1 year to 25% if the seizure occurred after that age. In addition, 25–50% of recurrent febrile seizures are not preceded by a fever. Instead, the seizure is the first sign of an illness (usually viral) and the fever comes later.

The vast majority of children with febrile seizures do not have seizures without fever after age 6. Risk factors for later epilepsy include (1) abnormal development before the febrile seizure, (2) complex febrile seizures (seizures lasting longer than 15 minutes, more than one seizure in 24 hours, or movements restricted to one side), and (3) a history of seizures without fever in a parent or a brother or sister. If none of these risk factors are present, the chances of later epilepsy are similar to that of the general population; if one risk factor is present, the chances of later epilepsy are 2.5%; if two or more risk factors are present, the chances of later epilepsy are 5 to more than 10%. Very rarely, febrile seizures that last more than 30 minutes may cause scar tissue in the temporal lobe and chronic epilepsy.

Febrile seizures cannot be prevented by baths, by applying cool cloths to the child's head or body, or by using fever-reducing medications such as acetaminophen (Tylenol) or ibuprofen (Advil, Motrin). Studies provide evidence against the intuition of most parents and pediatricians, but the results seem clear. Acetaminophen and ibuprofen are safe and can help a feverish child feel better, but they do not prevent febrile seizures. Aspirin should not be given to young children.

Most children with recurrent febrile seizures do not require daily antiepileptic drug therapy. Children who have had more than three febrile seizures or prolonged febrile seizures, or who have seizures when they have no fever, are often treated with daily medication. Diazepam, if given by mouth (Valium) or rectum (Diastat) at the time of fever, can prevent recurrent febrile seizures. However, the effective oral dose can cause irritability, insomnia, or other troublesome side effects that last for days. Prolonged febrile seizures can be terminated with rectal diazepam or buccal (between lip and gum) midazolam.

Benign Rolandic Epilepsy

> We heard a thud from Timmy's room one night. We rushed in and saw him on the floor, having a whole body seizure. The next day, the pediatrician asked if Timmy had ever had any tingling or jerking movements. We were shocked when Timmy said yes, sometimes his tongue would tingle or his cheek would jerk. The doctor did an EEG and said it was "rolandic epilepsy," and said that Timmy didn't have to be treated. That's what we wanted to hear. He had one other, milder seizure a few months later. It woke us up but he couldn't talk because the side of his mouth was twitching and he was drooling. It's been 5 years now, and except for a few tingles and twitches, Timmy has been doing great.

Benign rolandic epilepsy (benign epilepsy with centrotemporal spikes [BECTS]) is a common childhood seizure syndrome, with seizures beginning between 2 and 13 years of age. A hereditary factor is often present. The most characteristic attack is a partial motor (twitching) or a sensory (numbness or tingling sensation) seizure involving either side of the face or tongue (the side can change from one seizure to the next) that may cause garbled speech, but tonic-clonic seizures may occur. Seizures usually occur during sleep or in the transition into or out of sleep. Although the seizures are often infrequent or may occur in clusters of several a week followed by none for 6 months, some patients need medication. These include children who, in addition to the typical seizure disorder, have daytime or recurrent tonic-clonic seizures, a learning or cognitive disorder, or multiple seizures at night that cause tiredness in the morning. The seizures are easily controlled with low to moderate doses of a drug for partial epilepsy. If a drug is needed, it can almost always be discontinued by age 15, when the epilepsy spontaneously resolves.

The EEG shows spikes over the central and temporal regions (Fig. 3.1), which become more frequent during sleep. The abundance of epilepsy waves contrasts with the infrequent mild seizures. Siblings or close relatives may have the same EEG pattern during childhood without seizures.

Juvenile Myoclonic Epilepsy

> I have always had these little jerks, ever since I was 12, but I assumed everybody had them. They never really bothered me until a big one made me fall. I was put on medication for a few years, and then the drugs were stopped. During college, whenever I stayed up all night or drank too much, the next day I would get lots of jerks, and sometimes a big seizure right after the jerks.

Juvenile myoclonic epilepsy (JME) is a common epilepsy syndrome, defined by myoclonic seizures (jerks) with or without tonic-clonic or absence seizures. The EEG usually shows a pattern of spikes-and-waves or polyspikes-and-waves. CT and MRI scans of the brain are normal and typically are not needed.

Seizures usually begin shortly before or after puberty, or sometimes in early adulthood. Seizures are most frequent in the early morning, soon after awakening. Persons with JME often have seizures that may be triggered by flickering light, such as strobe lights at dances, TV, video games, or light shining through trees or reflecting off of ocean waves or snow. These are called photosensitive seizures. Myoclonic seizures also may be provoked by factors such as reading, decision-making or calculations (see pages 30–31). The intellectual functions of persons with JME are usually the same as those in the general population, although there may be some problems with "executive functions" such as planning and abstract reasoning.

In most cases the seizures are well controlled with medication, but the disorder is usually lifelong. Valproate is the treatment of choice, although many patients, especially women may not tolerate side effects. (See Appendix B for a summary of drug treatments of myoclonic, absence,

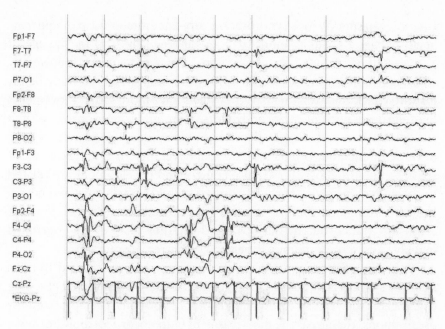

FIGURE 3.1: An EEG reveals centrotemporal spikes (abnormal epilepsy waves recorded over the central and temporal regions) from a boy with benign rolandic epilepsy. The labels on the left side of the figure indicate the area of the brain from which each recording was obtained.

and tonic-clonic seizures.) This syndrome may have a genetic basis, but in most patients no first-degree relatives are affected.

Infantile Spasms

> At first I thought Chris was just having the little body jerks when he was moved or startled, like my other children had when they were infants. But then I knew something was wrong. The jerks became more violent, and his tiny body spasmed forward and his arms flew apart. They only lasted a few seconds but started to occur in groups lasting a few minutes. So hard to see a young baby having these things.

Infantile spasms (West's syndrome), a very uncommon form of epilepsy, begin between 3 and 12 months of age and usually stop by the age of 2–4 years. The seizures, or spasms, consist of a sudden jerk followed by stiffening. With some spells, the arms are flung out as the body bends forward ("jackknife seizures"). Other spells have more subtle movements limited to the neck or other body parts. A brain disorder or injury, such as birth trauma with oxygen deprivation, precedes the seizures in 60% of these infants, but others have normal development until the onset of spasms. The prognosis for seizure control and development are related to the underlying cause of the seizures, the child's intellectual and neurological development before seizures begin (the better the condition at that time, the better the outlook), and whether seizures are controlled quickly. The sooner therapy is begun, the better the outcome.

A hormonal therapy as well as antiepileptic drugs are used to treat infantile spasms. Some experts recommend a trial of an antiepileptic drug (e.g., vigabatrin, valproate, topiramate) before hormonal therapy, but most use hormonal therapy as the first treatment (adrenocorticotropic hormone [ACTH]). ACTH is made by the pituitary gland and stimulates the adrenal glands to make cortisol. If the first treatment, whether ACTH, vigabatrin, or another antiepileptic drug such as topiramate, does not control the seizures within a week, another therapy should be considered.

In countries where it is available,* vigabatrin (Sabril) is often used as the initial therapy because it is safe for short-term use and effective. Vigabatrin is especially effective in children with tuberous sclerosis (a disorder affecting the brain, skin, heart, and other organs).

In the United States, ACTH is often used as the first therapy. ACTH is must be given as an injection, once a day for the first several weeks, then every other day for approximately 3 months. ACTH stops seizures in more than half of children with infantile spasms. The dosage is highest during the first week and then usually lowered gradually. Side effects depend on the dose used, the duration of therapy, and the baby's sensitivity. Complications are due to the effects of excessive cortisol, a steroid hormone: severe irritability, insomnia, increased appetite, weight gain, high blood pressure, kidney problems, redistribution of body fat (face and trunk fatter; arms and legs thinner), increased risk of infection

*Although not available in the United States, vigabatrin can be obtained from Canada, Mexico, and many other countries (see Chapter 11).

or gastrointestinal bleeding, increased blood glucose (hyperglycemia) and sodium (hypernatremia), and decreased potassium (hypokalemia). The benefits of ACTH outweigh the side effects for most children. If the spasms stopped with ACTH therapy, the treatment course is completed and another antiepileptic drug is often prescribed.

Even when the spasms stop, other seizure types often develop later on. Even without any treatment, infantile spasms will stop in more than 90% of children by the age of 5 years. Untreated children often have frequent spasms for many years, however, and later have partial or generalized seizures or other epileptic syndromes. One fifth of the cases of infantile spasms develop Lennox-Gastaut syndrome.

Lennox-Gastaut Syndrome

The first time I heard Tommy's diagnosis, Lennox-Gastaut syndrome, the words had no meaning. I went to the Internet, I was in tears within minutes. It sounded totally hopeless; there was no future. Ten years later, Tommy's seizures are under much better control. He loves school (special ed classes), has lots of friends, is an incredibly important part of our family, and gives us all great pleasure. He can almost beat me at tennis!

The parent of a child with Lennox-Gastaut syndrome needs lots of patience. Kathy has been on every medication, many of them three or four times. Nothing has ever controlled the seizures well. As the doctors kept going up on the doses, she would undergo terrible personality changes, turn into a zombie, or look drunk. We have finally come to accept the seizures and her mental handicaps. We also have part-time help at home so that we and our other kids can have a more normal life. As we let go of some our unrealistic hopes and accepted Kathy for who she is, disappointment changed to joy.

The Lennox-Gastaut syndrome is serious but uncommon. It is defined by three features: difficult-to-control seizures, mental retardation, and a slow spike-and-wave pattern on the EEG. The seizures usually begin between 1 and 6 years of age, but can begin later. The syndrome involves some combination of tonic, atypical absence, myoclonic, and tonic-clonic seizures that are usually resistant to medications. Most children with the Lennox-Gastaut syndrome have mild to severe intellectual impairment and behavioral problems that result from a combination of the neurologic injury, seizures, and antiepileptic drugs.

The course of the seizures varies greatly. Some children achieve good, although rarely complete, seizure control. Others continue to have drop attacks, atypical absence, partial and tonic-clonic seizures. The intellectual and behavioral development of children often parallels seizure control—the better the control, the better the development. Frequent seizures, especially those that cause falls, often lead to head injuries and the need for high doses of several AEDs. Both of these factors can increase the disability. Lennox-Gastaut syndrome usually persists into adulthood, and affected persons often need to live in a residential (adult foster care) group home when their parents are no longer able to care for them.

Medications that are useful for controlling the seizures of patients with Lennox-Gastaut syndrome include valproate, carbamazepine, clobazam (not in the United States), lamotrigine, topiramate, and zonisamide. Felbamate is effective, but it has a relatively high risk of life-threatening blood or liver disorders, and patients must be monitored with frequent blood tests.

For patients with poorly controlled seizures, it is best to avoid high doses of multiple antiepileptic drugs because they may intensify the behavioral, social, and intellectual problems. It may be better to tolerate slightly more frequent seizures to have a more alert and attentive child whose quality of life is much improved. Vagus nerve stimulation or corpus callosotomy (see Chapter 13) can help some patients. Because it has lower risks, we recommend vagus nerve stimulation before callosotomy.

Reflex Epilepsies

Reflex epilepsies are provoked by specific triggers, usually in the environment. Most reflex epilepsies are primary generalized epilepsy, although some are due to partial epilepsy. The most common form is

> It was only later that I realized he was sitting under a flickering fluorescent light when he had his first seizure. All three of his seizures have happened with flashing or flickering lights. Once he had a seizure while driving through a shaded area where the light flickers through the leaves and branches. Now we give him dark sunglasses, and he keeps his head down in this setting.

photosensitive epilepsy—a generalized epilepsy—which often begins in childhood and is often outgrown before adulthood. Flashing lights can elicit absence, myoclonic seizures or tonic-clonic seizures. People with photosensitive epilepsies should try to avoid flashing lights, but this is not always easy as some common settings can be provocative, such as a disco lights or police cars. For some people, certain rates of blinking (-12–18 Hz) or colors are mostlikely to provoke seizures. Certain video games can provoke seizures, but this is very uncommon (see Chapter 17).

Other environmental triggers in reflex epilepsy include sounds such as a loud startling noise, a certain type of music, or a person's voice; doing arithmetic; reading; and certain movements, such as writing. Internal triggers such as thinking about specific topics or experiencing an emotion can also provoke seizures. Because environmental triggers may be unavoidable or because nonreflex seizures also occur, many persons require treatment.

Temporal Lobe Epilepsy

> I get the strangest feeling; most of it can't be put into words. The whole world suddenly seems more real at first; it's as though everything becomes crystal clear. Then I feel as if I'm here but not here, kind of like being in a dream. It's as if I've lived through this exact moment many times before. I hear what people say, but they don't make sense. I know not to talk during the episode, since I just say foolish things. Sometimes I think I'm talking but later people tell me that I didn't say anything. It lasts a minute or two.

This description depicts some of the unusual features of temporal lobe seizures. Symptoms can be extremely varied, but certain patterns are common (see Chapter 2). The seizure experiences and sensations are often impossible to describe, even for eloquent adults. It can be extremely difficult to obtain an accurate picture of what children feel. There may be a mixture of different feelings, emotions, thoughts, and experiences, which may be strangely familiar or foreign. In some cases, a series of old memories resurfaces; in others, the person may feel as if everything— including his or her home and family—appears strange. Hallucinations of voices, music, people, smells, or tastes may occur.

Experiences during temporal lobe seizures vary in intensity and quality. Seizures may be so mild that the person barely notices or they may consume a person with fright, intellectual fascination, or occasionally, pleasure.

Dostoyevsky, the Russian novelist, had epilepsy and gave vivid accounts of temporal lobe seizures in his novel *The Idiot*-for example:

> He remembered that during his epileptic fits, or rather immediately preceding them, he had always experienced a moment or two when his whole heart, and mind, and body seemed to wake up with vigor and light; when he became filled with joy and hope, and all his anxieties seemed to be swept away for ever; these moments were but presentiments, as it were, of the one final second ... in which the fit came upon him. That second, of course, was inexpressible.

Complex partial seizures, most often with automatisms such as lip smacking and hand rubbing, represent the most common seizure type. Three quarters of people with temporal lobe epilepsy also have simple partial seizures, and half have tonic-clonic seizures at some time. Some only have simple partial seizures.

Seizures usually begin in the deeper portions of the temporal lobe, in limbic areas, which control emotions and memory (see Fig. A1.3C). Some individuals have short-term memory problems, especially if seizures have occurred for more than 5 years or there have been multiple tonic-clonic seizures.

In most cases, the seizures can be well controlled with antiepileptic drugs. If drugs are not effective, temporal lobectomy surgery can often control seizures (see Chapter 13). Vagus nerve stimulation may also be beneficial when temporal lobectomy is not recommended or has failed.

Frontal Lobe Epilepsy

> My head starts jerking toward the right side. I try, but can't stop it. Then my right hand goes up and my head turns toward the hand. I may just stay in that position for half a minute and it's over, or it can become a grand mal seizure.

> Usually I don't get any warning, I just have tonic-clinic seizures. Occasionally I get a momentary warning of a strange feeling in my head.

> I spend the night watching Molly sleep sometimes. She will have 5 or 10 seizures in a single night. They are short, usually less than 20 seconds. Her body rocks, like she is adjusting her position in the bed, and then she may start to make these kicking movements with her legs, like she is riding a bicycle. She may not have any more seizures for a month or two.

> Craig has had the same giggles for more than a decade. Now they occur mainly when he is exercising or stressed. He makes a weird smirk and giggles for a few seconds. He can cover it up and the kids don't know. If he misses his medications, he can have a bigger seizure.

Frontal lobe epilepsy is the second most common type of partial epilepsy. The frontal lobes are large (see Fig. A1.1A, B) and have motor (movement), cognitive, and behavioral functions. When motor areas are affected, abnormal movements (jerks, stiffness) can occur on the opposite side of the body. Motor area seizures can also result in weakness or the inability to use certain muscles. Seizures arising in other cognitive or behavioral areas can cause psychic, autonomic, or other symptoms like temporal lobe epilepsy. Symptoms may only occur when the seizure discharge spreads to other areas.

In comparison with temporal lobe complex partial seizures, those beginning in the frontal lobe tend to be shorter (usually less than 1 minute), are less likely to be followed by confusion or tiredness, more often occur in a cluster or series, and are more likely to include strange automatisms such as bicycling movements, screaming, or sexual activity. A person may remain fully aware during a frontal lobe seizure while having wild movements of the arms and legs. Because of their strange nature, frontal lobe seizures can be misdiagnosed as nonepileptic seizures (see Chapter 8). The clinical features can suggest whether seizures begin in the frontal or temporal lobes, but the EEG during a seizure often provides the best information. An MRI showing an abnormality provides strong evidence for where the seizure begins.

Frontal lobe seizures are treated with medications for partial seizures, but may also be treated surgically or with vagus nerve stimulation (see Chapter 13).

Rare Epilepsy Syndromes

Generalized Epilepsy Febrile Seizures-Plus (GEFS+)

GEFS+ is a recently described genetic syndrome in which the range of clinical features and varieties of chromosomal abnormalities grows as we learn more. Most patients have problems in the DNA that codes for the proteins in sodium channels in cell membranes. The altered proteins change neuronal excitability and predispose to seizures. There is often more than one person in the family affected with some combination of febrile or afebrile seizures. Some patients have only simple febrile seizures that end before age 6 years, while others can have febrile seizures that are prolonged or recur after age 6. Other types include absence, myoclonic, atonic, and partial seizures. Some patients have very benign courses, while in others the seizures are poorly controlled, such as severe myoclonic epilepsy of infancy (Dravet syndrome; see below). A test for some of the common DNA mutations can be done by Athena Diagnostics.

Severe Myoclonic Epilepsy of Infancy
(SMEI or Dravet Syndrome)

SMEI typically begins in the first year of life, affecting infants who were usually developmentally normal until seizures begin. Seizures may be prolonged and are often provoked by fever, especially during the first several years of the disorder. Initially, generalized or unilateral clonic seizures occur but are followed by myoclonic and partial seizures. Developmental delays and other neurologic problems such as unsteadiness often develop. The seizures are often difficult to control and lifelong. Some patients have abnormalities in their sodium channel genes that can be tested by Athena Diagnostics.

SMEI should be distinguished from Lennox-Gastaut syndrome and Doose syndrome. The history of febrile clonic seizures helps distinguish SMEI patients from those with Lennox-Gastaut syndrome. The EEG in SMEI often shows features of both generalized and localized (partial) epilepsy waves. Although febrile convulsive seizures may occur myoclonic-astatic epilepsy (Doose syndrome) as well as SMEI, those with Doose syndrome do not show localized epilepsy waves and do not develop partial seizures.

Myoclonic-Astatic Epilepsy of Early Childhood
(MAE or Doose Syndrome)

In MAE, myoclonic and drop (astatic) seizures almost always begin in an 18- to 50-month-old child who was developmentally normal until seizures began. Other seizure types include absence and tonic-clonic seizures. The course varies: some children outgrow their seizures and are developmentally normal, while others have developmental delays and persistent seizures.

Landau-Kleffner Syndrome

The Landau-Kleffner syndrome causes the loss of previously acquired language abilities (aquired aphasia) and epilepsy activity and affects boys more than girls. Typically, a child between 3 and 8 years of age suddenly or gradually experiences language problems, with or without seizures. It usually affects auditory comprehension (understanding spoken language) most, but speaking ability can also (or solely) be affected. Simple partial motor and tonic-clonic are infrequent, often nocturnal, and easily controlled with medications.

The EEG during sleep is the key to the diagnosis. A normal EEG, especially one done when the child is awake, does not rule out this disorder. Sleep activates the epilepsy waves, which may be localized over language areas or more generalized.

The boundaries of the Landau-Kleffner syndrome are imprecise. A variant may occur in some children in whom language function is delayed or never develops. The epilepsy waves likely contribute to or cause the language disorder.

Antiepileptic drugs are ineffective in treating the language disorder. Steroids may improve the EEG abnormalities and language problems. A type of epilepsy surgery, multiple subpial transections (see Chapter 13), can be helpful in selected cases.

Electrical Status Epilepticus of Slow Wave Sleep (ESES) or Continuous Spike and Wave in Slow Wave Sleep (CSWS)

This rare syndrome affects children with a regression of language, memory, and other cognitive and behavioral skills. Onset is most common between ages 5 and 7 years of age, with a slight male predominance. The key diagnostic feature is nearly continuous generalized (slow spike and wave discharges), or less often localized, epilepsy waves in non-rapid eye movement (REM) sleep. The group includes a spectrum of children. One third have abnormalities on MRI such as decreased brain size (atrophy) or malformations of cortical development. The prognosis for seizure control and development is variable. Seizures are often difficult to control with antiepileptic drugs, and some patients respond well to steroids, as in Landau-Kleffner syndrome. Some centers use high doses of benzodiazepines for short periods.

Rasmussen's Syndrome

Rasmussen's syndrome usually begins between 14 months and 14 years of age and is associated with slowly progressive neurologic deterioration and simple partial and tonic-clonic seizures. Seizures are often the first problem. Epilepsia partialis continua—a prolonged seizure with jerking of one side—is also common and responds poorly to medication.

Although Rasmussen's syndrome is rarely fatal, its effects are devastating. Progressive weakness on one side (hemiparesis) and mental retardation are common, and language disorder (aphasia) often occurs if the language hemisphere is affected. Mild weakness of an arm or leg is the most common initial symptom besides seizures. Weakness and other neurologic problems often begin 1–3 years after the seizures start. Serial CT and MRI scans show a slow loss (atrophy) of brain substance. Rasmussen's syndrome is probably an autoimmune disorder (antibodies are produced against the body's own tissues) that may be triggered by a viral infection.

Treatment with antiepileptic drugs is disappointing. Steroids and other immune-modulating therapies such as gamma globulin or plasmapheresis may help. In children with severe loss of function in the involved hemisphere, a surgical procedure, functional hemispherectomy (see Chapter 13), can be successful.

Progressive Myoclonic Epilepsies

> After a few tonic-clonics, they started Avi on medication. Each drug worked for a while and then his body became immune to it. They tried more and more drugs, two or three at a time, and the seizures just became more frequent. The worst part was that Avi was slipping—he was changing. He was not as sharp and quick as he had been. We blamed the drugs, but it just got worse. Then came the little seizures that would cause his speech to sputter and hesitate and his mind to turn on and off, like someone was taking a light switch and flicking it up and down.

Progressive myoclonic epilepsies cause myoclonic and tonic-clonic seizures that are difficult to control and associated with deteriorating neurologic function. Seizures are often triggered by movement or sensory stimuli (sound, touch or visual). These epilepsies are rare and usually result from different hereditary metabolic disorders, but in some cases the cause remains unknown.

Antiepileptic drugs are of limited benefit. As the disorder progresses, drugs become less effective, and side effects may be more severe. In such cases, it is often worthwhile to avoid very high doses of multiple antiepi-leptic drugs. Drugs for myoclonic and generalized tonic-clonic seizures (see Chapter 12), such as valproate and zonisamide, are useful.

Mitochondrial Disorders

Mitochondria are the energy factories of the cell. Abnormalities in mitochondrial function cause metabolic disorders that affect different parts of the body, including muscle and brain. Several mitochondrial disorders cause myoclonic, absence, and tonic-clonic seizures and other neurologic problems such as stroke-like episodes, hearing loss, dementia, headaches, vomiting, unsteadiness, and problems with exercise. Mitochondrial disorders are diagnosed by testing blood and spinal fluid for levels of certain chemicals. The most definitive diagnostic test is a muscle biopsy to assess mitochondrial enzyme activity; if abnormal, the mitochondrial DNA should then be examined for mutations. A commercial test (Athena Diagnositics) can test for some specific genetic disorders from a blood sample.

Hypothalamic Hamartoma and Epilepsy

Small tumors in the base of the brain that affect the hypothalamus (see Fig. A1.1C) can cause early puberty, partial seizures with laughing as a frequent feature, and irritability and aggression between the seizures. Simple and complex partial and secondary generalized tonic-clonic seizures can occur. Affected individuals are often short and have mild abnormalities in their physical features (dysmorphisms). MRI is necessary for diagnosis. Surgery can control seizures in some cases. Antiepileptic drugs can also be beneficial, as can drugs aimed at hormonal and behavioral problems, if needed.

4 | Causes of Epilepsy

A seizure is a symptom of an underlying process in the brain that can have many different causes. Epilepsy is a disorder rather than a "disease." Thus, there are many causes of seizures and epilepsy. Anything that injures the brain or disrupts the electrical or chemical balance can cause epilepsy. A detailed history, neurologic examination, and MRI sometimes reveal a cause for the recurrent seizures (symptomatic epilepsy). In rare cases, the history, exam, and imaging are normal, but several family members have epilepsy and a genetic cause is suspected. In many cases the cause remains unknown.

The cause of epilepsy is often incorrectly identified. For example, many children have a history of "a difficult delivery" or have their first seizure shortly after a vaccination. Similarly, many children and adults have their first seizure within weeks or months of a mild head injury (loss of consciousness for less than 10 minutes). In such cases, although it is natural to assume a causal relationship, extensive studies strongly support coincidence. People have a strong desire to identify a cause—this can lead to the right answer, but also to a wrong "answer."

Is There a Known Cause?

Symptomatic epilepsy refers to epilepsy with an identified cause other than genetics. Causes include severe head injury, scar tissue, problems of brain development, stroke, meningitis, and others. The cause is typically documented by clinical history (for example, head trauma with a 2-hour loss of consciousness), or neuroimaging (MRI or CT) reveals the abnormality. Partial or generalized epilepsy can be symptomatic.

Idiopathic epilepsy occurs without known cause. Most cases are primary generalized epilepsies, occurring in an otherwise normal person. In most cases, genetic factors are thought to lower seizure threshold. The person usually has no other disabilities.

Cryptogenic epilepsy refers to cases without sufficient information to determine if it is a symptomatic or idiopathic type. In most of the cryptogenic cases, a cause is suspected but cannot be identified. Cases of partial epilepsy without known cause are considered cryptogenic.

Partial Versus Generalized Epilepsies

The epilepsies are divided into two broad categories—partial and generalized—based on the clinical and EEG features. Partial epilepsies result from some localized brain disorder. In contrast, generalized seizures affect the brain more diffusely, involving wide areas of both sides at seizure onset. For many patients there is a fundamental difference in the biology of partial and generalized epilepsies. Partial seizures result from an identified (symptomatic) or suspected (cryptogenic) disorder affecting one or more localized brain areas. In patients with generalized epilepsy, genetic factors are suspected, even if no one else in the family has epilepsy. Some evidence suggests that these genes may control cellular structures such as ion channels and neurotransmitter receptors. However, the picture is complex. For example, hereditary factors and ion channel dysfunction can be involved in partial epilepsy. Also, generalized epilepsies may be "activated" by causes such as head injury.

Kindling: A Model of Partial Epilepsy

Patients often ask why there may be an interval of years between a brain injury and the first seizure. There is no single or simple answer to how epilepsy develops—the process of epileptogenesis. The kindling model provides insights. If an area of an animal's brain is stimulated once a day with a small electrical current, initially there may be no changes. After a week, there may be a small, local storm of electrical activity after the stimulation. After several weeks the storm may spread to neighboring areas and the animal may have symptoms such as facial grimacing or blank staring. As the stimulation is repeated, the electrical storms and seizure symptoms become more intense, eventually causing a tonic-clonic seizure. Finally, in some animals, spontaneous seizures occur—that is, without the electrical stimulation. Thus, a "fire" has been "kindled" in the brain. Moving up the phylogenetic tree—for example, from rats to baboons—the "kindling" process proceeds more slowly.

Of course, kindling experiments have never been done in humans. But the similarity between the patterns of seizures, the EEG activity, and the changes found in the brains of kindled animals and in patients with partial epilepsy suggests that kindling occurs in humans. Thus, a brain injury triggers abnormal electrical currents, which may progress over months or years to cause seizures.

Channelopathies: A Model of Primary Generalized Epilepsy?

Ion channels regulate the flow of charged molecules across cell membranes. These channels are of vital importance in electrically active nerve and muscle cells. Genetic changes in the structure to these complex proteins—even the substitution of a one amino acid for another at a critical site—can disrupt the fine balance of nerve cell excitability and lead to recurrent seizures. These disorders of ion channels, or channelopathies, are the most commonly recognized genetic cause of generalized epilepsy.

Most ion channel disorders occur in large families where many members have epilepsy. The EEG of those patients has the classic generalized three to five per second (Hz) spike-and-wave discharges (Fig. 9.4). However, most patients with generalized epilepsy do not have close relatives with epilepsy. However, these patients show similar EEG findings, suggesting that they may also have ion channel abnormalities.

Causes of Partial Epilepsy

Scientific studies of populations (epidemiologic studies) have identified many factors that cause epilepsy. Table 4.1 lists the major risk factors for epilepsy.

Table 4.1. Causes of Epilepsy

Factors Associated with 10-Fold or Greater Risk of Epilepsy

Infants with seizures in the first month of life

Head injury that causes one or more of the following:

> Loss of consciousness >30 minutes

> Significant memory impairment after the injury

> Abnormalities such as weakness or impaired coordination

> Skull fracture

Infections

> Meningitis

> Encephalitis

> Cerebral abscess

Brain tumors

Cerebral palsy

Mental retardation

Alzheimer's disease

Complicated (complex) febrile seizures

Stroke

Blood vessel malformations in the brain

> Arteriovenous malformations

> Cavernous angiomas

Alcohol abuse

Factors Associated with Less Than 10-Fold Risk of Epilepsy

Use of illegal drugs

Family history of epilepsy or febrile seizures

Multiple sclerosis

Seizures occurring within days after head injury ("early posttraumatic seizures")

There are many other disorders that affect the brain, either primarily or as part of a more widespread problem that also causes epilepsy. These include autism, metabolic disorders (such as mito-chondrial, amino acid and storage disorders), chromosomal disorders (such as trisomy 21 [Down syndrome], fragile X, ring chromosome 20), and neurocutaneous disorders (neurologic and skin involvement; such as tuberous sclerosis and neurofibromatosis).

Epidemiologic studies have failed to establish a clear relationship between vaccination and epilepsy. In some cases, however, vaccination can cause a fever that provokes a febrile convulsion. Similarly, mild head injury, such as a concussion with loss of consciousness for less than 10–15 minutes is not a cause of epilepsy (Fig. 4.1).

Hereditary Influences and Epilepsy

Hereditary (genetic) factors are important in some cases of epilepsy. When epilepsy develops at a young age, there is an increased risk of epilepsy among the brothers and sisters and the affected person's children. Genetic factors are more common in primary generalized epilepsy than in partial epilepsy.

Among patients with primary generalized epilepsy and generalized spike-and-waves on the EEG, the risk of epilepsy in a sibling is approximately 4%. When a child with absence or tonic-clonic seizures has generalized spike-and-waves and one of that child's brothers or sisters also has the spike-and-wave abnormality, another child in the family has an 8% risk of developing epilepsy. When a parent and a child have primary generalized epilepsy, there is a 10% risk that the parent's other children will have isolated seizures or epilepsy.

Heredity may influence the likelihood that a person will develop partial epilepsy after experiencing a cause of seizures, such as severe head injury. The rate of epilepsy is higher among family members of people who develop epilepsy with cerebral palsy than among the relatives of people who do not. Benign rolandic epilepsy is a partial epilepsy syndrome with a genetic component.

The children of parents with epilepsy also have an increased risk. By age 25 years, a child of a parent with epilepsy has a 6% chance of having an unprovoked seizure compared with 1–2% in the general

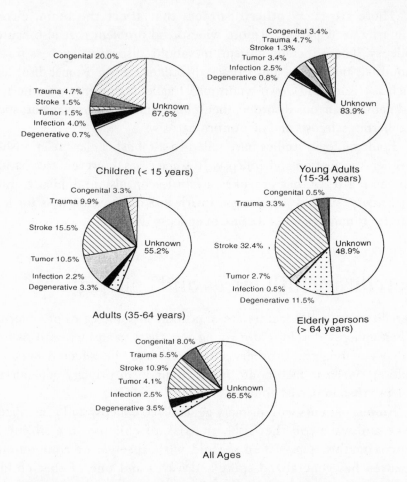

Congenital 20.0%
Trauma 4.7%
Stroke 1.5%
Tumor 1.5%
Infection 4.0%
Degenerative 0.7%
Unknown 67.6%

Children (< 15 years)

Congenital 3.4%
Trauma 4.7%
Stroke 1.3%
Tumor 3.4%
Infection 2.5%
Degenerative 0.8%
Unknown 83.9%

Young Adults (15-34 years)

Congenital 3.3%
Trauma 9.9%
Stroke 15.5%
Tumor 10.5%
Infection 2.2%
Degenerative 3.3%
Unknown 55.2%

Adults (35-64 years)

Congenital 0.5%
Trauma 3.3%
Stroke 32.4%
Tumor 2.7%
Infection 0.5%
Degenerative 11.5%
Unknown 48.9%

Elderly persons (> 64 years)

Congenital 8.0%
Trauma 5.5%
Stroke 10.9%
Tumor 4.1%
Infection 2.5%
Degenerative 3.5%
Unknown 65.5%

All Ages

FIGURE 4.1: The percentage of cases of epilepsy resulting from various causes, shown for persons of all ages and different age groups. (From Hauser, WA: Seizure disorders: The changes with age. Epilepsia (Suppl 4)22:s6–s14, 1992, with permission.)

population. Epilepsy is more common among the children of women with epilepsy than among the children of men with epilepsy.

In cases where heredity is important, a single gene or several genes may be the determining factor. More than 12 epilepsy syndromes are linked to specific genes, but each one is uncommon or rare.

5 | The First Seizure

> I woke up in the ambulance with an oxygen mask on my face and had no idea what had happened. I tried to get up, to get away. People were asking me if I knew my name, but my head felt so heavy and I was really confused. The side of my tongue was throbbing in pain. Slowly I understood more, they said I had had a seizure? I am 40 years old and there's never been anything wrong with me. Why did this happen? What does this mean?

The first seizure is terrifying; its emotional trauma can be devastating. If it is a tonic-clonic seizure, witnesses are usually more shaken than the patient. But the real fear comes after the seizure ends—what is the underlying cause? Will there be another? Is this the start of some terrible affliction? Are drugs needed? Will the medicines need to be taken forever? Knowledge of epilepsy can reduce the fear about the risk of having another seizure as well as the anxiety and feelings of vulnerability about the unpredictability of if, and when, another seizure may occur. Other concerns arise from the real and perceived stigma associated with "epilepsy," possibility of physical injury or loss of driving privileges, employment issues, embarrassment, and the effects of antiepileptic drugs (AEDs) on a future pregnancy. Remember—the vast majority of people who have a single seizure do extremely well!

After a first seizure, the person should be evaluated, often in an emergency room, to exclude uncommon but potentially life-threatening problems such as meningitis, stroke, or metabolic disorders. Examination by a doctor, blood tests, and neuroimaging (CT or MRI) tests will rapidly eliminate these dangerous and treatable causes. For most patients, these tests are either normal or reveal a benign problem that may have caused the seizure.

Risk of Recurrence

After a single, unprovoked convulsive seizure, the risk of at least one more seizure is approximately 50%; recurrences are most likely to occur within a year. If someone experiences two seizures, the chances of having a third one are about 80%. The risk of recurrence after a first seizure is roughly twice as high for people with a known brain injury or other type of brain abnormality (symptomatic epilepsy) than it is for those with no known injury (cryptogenic and idiopathic epilepsies). It is also higher for those with partial seizures or an abnormal EEG.

Of people who had a brain injury in the past (such as head trauma or brain infection), those who had a seizure at the time of the injury are more likely to develop epilepsy than those who did not. People with abnormalities on neurologic examination are at slightly greater risk of a second seizure than those with normal results.

The EEG also helps predict recurrence after a single seizure. People with abnormalities characteristic of epilepsy (epilepsy waves; such as spike-and-wave discharges, spikes, or sharp waves) have approximately twice the chance of having another seizure than do people with normal EEGs or with other kinds of abnormalities such as mild slowing (see Chapter 9 and Table 19.1). Epilepsy waves on the EEG is most important in predicting recurrent seizures in people with no history of brain injury or abnormality.

We are not sure whether epilepsy in a family member increases the risk of recurrence after a person's first seizure. Most studies have found either no increase or only a slightly increased recurrence rate.

To Treat or Not to Treat?

> Everyone told me I had a big seizure. In the emergency room they did some tests, and said everything checked out ok. The ER doc told me they don't usually prescribe medication after a single seizure, but recommended that I follow up with a neurologist. Later, I read on the Internet about seizures, and am pretty sure I have had smaller ones. I went to the neurologist and told him about these other "feelings"; he recommended a prolonged EEG, and said I might need to take medication.

This discussion of first seizures applies only to tonic-clonic seizures. As a rule, when a single absence seizure is reported and confirmed on EEG, the child usually has had many other staring spells that were not reported, and treatment is usually recommended. Similarly, with partial seizures, a person commonly may have had several partial seizures, but one relatively prominent episode or a convulsion leads to medical attention. If the diagnosis of a partial seizure is uncertain and the neuroimaging and EEG studies are normal or do not suggest epilepsy, most doctors would not prescribe an AED. If a partial seizure has occurred, however, many doctors would consider treatment because there is a high probability of recurrence. One exception is with benign rolandic epilepsy; many experts may not recommend treatment even after a tonic-clonic seizure (see Chapter 3).

There is no simple answer as to whether or not to treat a single tonic-clonic seizure. The chance of seizure recurrence is 40–50% depending on the patient, the seizure type, and the circumstances surrounding the seizure. The chances of a second seizure are lower if the following are normal: neurologic examination, neuroimaging studies, and EEG. Other factors supporting a decision not to treat include (1) provocation factors such as sleep deprivation or excessive alcohol intake before the seizure that can be eliminated, (2) seizure occurrence during sleep (a second seizure will more likely occur in sleep), and (3) lack of a family history of epilepsy. Table 19.1 shows the risk of a recurrent seizure during the 2 years after a seizure in children, based on whether the EEG shows epilepsy waves and whether the neurologic examination was abnormal. The risk factors in adults are similar.

Some decisions about treatment are more difficult than others. A 10-year-old child with a single seizure during sleep who has a normal examination, MRI scan, and EEG probably should probably not receive medication. In contrast, treatment is advisable for a 30-year-old woman who has a single daytime convulsion, scar tissue on MRI, and abundant epilepsy activity on the EEG who drives hundreds of miles each week in her job. Most patients fall between these two extremes. Treatment decisions should consider the chances that another seizure will occur, patient's lifestyle, side effects of the medications, and the plan for discontinuing medications if seizures do not recur after a period of time.

The decision to use an AED can create other questions. In about half of patients, the first drug is replaced by another drug because of more seizures or side effects. Should the person drive immediately after medications are started, or only after the level of the drug in the blood reaches a certain level, or after a set period of time, such as 3–12 months? If no seizures occur during treatment, how long should treatment last? If the person is seizure-free for a year or two, is it safe to continue driving when the drugs are tapered off and discontinued? Although laws and regulations vary in each state, many of these questions are not clearly addressed by state laws and fall into the "grey zone" of judgment.

6 | Prognosis of Epilepsy

Remission of Epilepsy and Risk of Recurrence

After epilepsy is diagnosed and effective therapy is prescribed, approximately two thirds of people will be seizure-free for 5 years. The longer the time between seizures, the greater the chance of permanent remission (seizure freedom). Twenty years after the diagnosis of epilepsy, approximately three quarters of people will have been seizure-free for at least 5 years. If seizures stop, they usually do so within the first 2 years after diagnosis. The longer the time that people continue to have seizures after epilepsy is diagnosed, however, the lower the chances of a remission. Nevertheless, even people with intractable epilepsy (seizures that cannot be controlled with tolerable medication doses) may later become seizure-free.

People with primary generalized seizures, especially tonic-clonic seizures, have a better chance of remission than those with other kinds. Also, those who are younger when the diagnosis of epilepsy is made are more likely to stop having seizures than older people. The remission rate is also higher if the person has no brain injury or abnormality and if his or her neurologic examination is normal.

The role of the EEG in predicting whether epilepsy will go into remission varies by epilepsy syndrome. The characteristic EEG pattern of centrotemporal spikes (see Fig. 3.1) in benign rolandic epilepsy virtually guarantees remission by age 15 years. People with the generalized spike-and-wave EEG pattern characteristic of primary generalized epilepsy are less likely to become seizure-free than those with a normal EEG. This difference partly reflects patients with juvenile myoclonic epilepsy, who often have such EEG abnormalities and have low remission rates. The predictive value of other epilepsy wave patterns is uncertain.

People with epilepsy who have been seizure-free for 5 years may later have seizures again. Overall, about 1.5% of people who have been seizure-free for 5 years have another seizure. Such a relapse is more likely in people with complex partial seizures and those who are older than 20 years.

There is some risk of relapse after AEDs are discontinued, but they may also play a role in the remission of epilepsy. More than 100 years ago, the English neurologist Sir William Gowers suggested that "seizures beget seizures." That is, once you have one seizure, you are more likely to have another simply because your brain "learns" how to have a seizure. This may partly result from the kindling process (see Chapter 4). Although his concept remains unproved, some evidence suggests that he was right, at least in some cases. In children, this may be true only after 10 or more tonic-clonic seizures have occurred. The longer someone remains seizure-free while taking AEDs, the better chance he or she has of remaining seizure-free when the medication is stopped. Just as the brain learns to have seizures, it may also "forget" to have seizures. AEDs may enhance the forgetting process by controlling seizures. This effect of AEDs, however, is unproven.

Most people who are seizure-free for 2–4 years can stop taking their medications without having further seizures. About 20–35% of children and 30–65% of adults will have seizures again after medication is withdrawn, however. Currently, most neurologists in the United States consider withdrawing AEDs after someone has been seizure-free for 1–2 years. In Europe and Canada, medication is often withdrawn after 6 months without seizures for children with a good outlook. Whether the person takes part in hazardous activities such as driving or swimming may influence the doctor's decision of when to withdraw an AED (see Chapter 19).

Chronic, Well-Controlled Epilepsy

Some patients remain seizure-free on AEDs, but when they attempt to come off their medications, seizures recur. In many cases, the recurrence is due to sleep deprivation, alcohol intake, or emotional stress. However, some of these factors may be difficult to eliminate. This group, approximately 20% of epilepsy patients, mainly includes people with partial epilepsy as well as primary generalized syndromes such as juvenile myoclonic epilepsy.

Medically Refractory Epilepsy

Among newly diagnosed patients with epilepsy, approximately 25%–30% do not come under control with AEDs—that is, medically refractory epilepsy. Risk factors for medically refractory epilepsy include partial epilepsy, more than one seizure type, abnormalities on neurologic examination or imaging studies, long duration of active epilepsy, and frequent seizures at onset.

What Happens to Untreated Epilepsy?

The natural history of untreated epilepsy is not well known. In some cases, epilepsy remits without treatment. No well-designed studies can answer the question of whether or not treatment, or early treatment, reduces the risk for chronic or medically refractory epilepsy. However, available evidence does not support that early treatment is critical to improving prognosis.

Associated Disorders

For many people, the disorders associated with epilepsy—such as depression, anxiety, and memory loss—are more disabling than the seizures. Many of these problems can result from multiple factors, including underlying brain disorder, recurrent (especially tonic-clonic) seizures, AEDs, and psychological issues. Prevention is an important strategy: controlling seizures with the lowest effective dose of a safe medication. A healthy diet and exercise can also help. Unfortunately, apart from frequent and severe seizures, we cannot predict which patients are at risk to develop cognitive and behavioral complications of epilepsy.

Epilepsy and Life Span

Although most patients with well-controlled epilepsy and normal neurological function have normal life spans, there is some risk to life associated with epilepsy.

Fatal Seizures

Convulsive (tonic-clonic) status epilepticus (see Chapter 2) is a medical emergency and may cause permanent injury or death if treatment is delayed or ineffective. Single seizures that impair consciousness are almost never life-threatening. Serious accidents and injuries, although rare, are increased for people with epilepsy. A tonic-clonic seizure may cause someone to fall in front of a train, for example, or to roll over in bed and suffocate. A complex partial seizure may cause a person to cross a busy street without caution. The most dangerous setting for someone with episodes of impaired consciousness is driving a motor vehicle, where a brief lapse can be deadly. Death from drowning is more common among people with epilepsy and can even occur in a bathtub.

Although seizures causing a fatal injury are *extremely rare*, prevention is the best medicine. People with seizures that impair consciousness or motor control should try to avoid situations that place them at risk. However, even activities of daily living—crossing streets, taking trains or subways—can be dangerous. There must be balance between safety and leading an active, productive, and enjoyable life (see Chapter 25). Nearly all people with epilepsy can achieve this balance.

Unexplained Death in Epilepsy

A rare condition, sudden unexplained death in epilepsy (SUDEP), occurs in young or middle-aged persons with epilepsy who die without a clearly defined cause. Many deaths occur in bed; about a third show evidence of a seizure near the time of death. They are often found lying on their stomach. Available evidence suggests that problems with breathing or the heart are most often responsible. Pulmonary (respiratory) problems include impaired breathing (apnea), increased fluid in the lungs (which impairs the exchange of oxygen and carbon dioxide), and possibly suffocation due to being face down on the bedding. Seizures can cause irregularities in the heart rhythm, which may rarely be life-threatening. In many cases, death probably occurs after the seizure has ended.

Safety precautions may reduce the chances of SUDEP:

1. Seizures, especially tonic-clonic seizures, should be well controlled. Patients should take their medications as prescribed and avoid provocative factors such as sleep deprivation and excess alcohol.
2. Adult patients* with a high likelihood of tonic-clonic seizures in sleep should be watched, if possible, or consider the use of a sleep monitor. These monitors can be simple ones that detect sound (a baby monitor) or more sophisticated ones that detect motion. For example, the MP5 is available from Easylink (easylinkuk.co.uk) for approximately $320. The MP5 is placed between the mattress and boxspring and can signal a caregiver in another room in the home when there is excessive movement. The MP5 can also be attached to an automated phone-dialing system to call neighbors or remote caregivers. For individuals at higher risk, it may be helpful to combine both sound and motion monitors.
3. Basic first aid should be provided, including rolling the person onto one side (see Chapter 10).

The risk of SUDEP for the average person with epilepsy is about 1 in 3000 per year. The risk for people with medically refractory epilepsy who have tonic-clonic seizures and take several AEDs is about 1 in 100–300 per year. Among all patients with epilepsy, SUDEP accounts for less than 2% of deaths. The risk is highest in young adults (ages 15–44), accounting for about 8% of deaths in this group.

---

*SUDEP is extremely rare in children with epilepsy.

II | Diagnosis and Treatment of Epilepsy

7 | Seizure- Provoking Factors

Many people with epilepsy can identify certain factors that increase their chances of having a seizure. Well-established factors include missed medication, sleep deprivation, excessive alcohol use, and the premenstrual period. Other factors such as emotional stress are commonly reported and very likely, but are difficult to prove. For some people, specific environmental factors such as flashing lights or startling noises can trigger seizures.

Many patients are surprised when missed medication or sleep deprivation leads to a breakthrough seizure because they had missed medication or gotten by on limited sleep at other times without having a seizure. However, more than one factor can contribute to the seizure susceptibility. For example, missing a single dose of medication may provoke a seizure in a person who also has not had enough sleep or in a woman around the time of her menstrual period, but not at other times. The risk of a breakthrough seizure is often related to the intensity and number of seizure-provoking factors. An unfortunately common example is partying by young adults who stay out late, drink excessively, and often forget their medication. In many other cases, we cannotdefine all of the variables that provoke (or control) seizures in an individual.

Seizure Calendar

A seizure calendar can help identify the type or frequency of seizures over time, the effect of different medications on seizure control, adverse effects of medications, and seizure-provoking factors. The most basic seizure calendar includes the date and time of the seizure, as well as the type of seizure. If a precipitating factor is suspected (e.g., lack of sleep, missed medication, stress, menstrual period), it should be noted. Try to record the medication, dosage, and blood levels of the drug. For women, it may be useful to track the relationship between seizures and the menstrual cycles (record the days of menstruation; ovulation occurs 14 days before menstruation).

Missed Medication

Missed medication is the most common cause of both breakthrough seizures and prolonged seizures (status epilepticus) that require emergency medical treatment. Status epilepticus is most likely to follow the abrupt discontinuation of one or more AEDs.

The most common and least harmful instance is occasionally missing a single dose. A missed dose is more common when an AED is taken three or four times per day rather than once or twice daily. When medication is taken once daily, however, one miss means the loss of a full day of medication, so it is more likely to cause seizures than if the medication is taken more often. Missing several doses in a row increases the likelihood of a breakthrough seizure. This sometimes happens when patients go away for a weekend, forget to pack their medication, and hope they can "get away without it for a few days."

Medications are missed for many reasons, and various preventive strategies can be employed. Always maintain a 1- to 2-week supply of medication. Those who order large quantities of AEDS by mail should have a spare 2- to 4-week supply. Keep extra medication in accessible places: at work, in the car, and in one's purse.* The school nurse or teacher should keep some for children. When going on a flight, try to

---

* Remember to "restock" the emergency supply so that it does not go out of date. This is especially important for emergency supplies that are stored in places (e.g., glove compartments of cars) that may become quite hot and shorten the shelf-life of a medication.

pack two separate supplies of medication: one in a carry-on bag and one for luggage that is checked. The hand-carried medications are "insurance" just in case the checked bag is misplaced or stolen.

Specific cues can help people remember to take all their medication. A person's daily pattern should help determine what time of day or activity would be a good point to stop and take the pills. Is there a specific time of day, such as 8 A.M. or 8 P.M.? Can the pills be taken with at breakfast and bedtime? Can the morning dosing be linked with brushing the teeth (rarely forgotten before leaving the house!), taking a shower, or some other bathroom activity? Make a special effort to remember to take the pills when the routine is interrupted, such as by sleeping late or skipping lunch. When a day is hectic and crazy, make taking the AED a priority. Pillboxes are very helpful to both organize medication by day of the week and time of day as well as help the person identify a missed dose (the pills are still in their compartment). Wristwatches and pillboxes can be programmed to remind one when the next dose is due.

Some persons with epilepsy decide to lower or discontinue their medication without a doctor's advice. This is dangerous! Rapid reduction or stopping an AED can cause withdrawal symptoms, including prolonged tonic-clonic seizures, even if they have never occurred before. Further, changes in one drug can alter the blood levels of other AED or medical drugs, and potentially cause a loss of effectiveness or serious side effects. An AED should never be stopped suddenly unless the doctor recommends it. If a doctor feels that it is unsafe to continue taking a medication (the patient gets a rash, for example), but if suddenly stopping the drug poses a risk of status epilepticus, he or she may prescribe another medication, or the person may be hospitalized when the drug is withdrawn.

The patient should always be comfortable discussing any issue with the doctor or nurse. If there are troublesome side effects, concerns about a known or planned pregnancy, fears that the AED is ineffective or worsening seizures—discuss them, don't stop medication on your own. If the doctor feels it is too dangerous or unwise to stop the drugs and the patient still feels strongly, consider a second opinion.

Refilling the Prescription

If the number of pills starts to get low and there are refills on the last prescription, get another supply from the pharmacy well before running out completely. If there are no refills left, the doctor will telephone the pharmacy if asked. Patients must *never wait until the last minute* to call the doctor or pharmacy.

Most doctors and clinics are available to speak with patients 24 hours a day. A patient will rarely need to call a doctor at 3 A.M. for a refill. Usually, the patient should call the doctor in the morning. If it is a weekend, it is best not to wait until Monday to call if it means running out of pills. If the doctor is unavailable and no other doctor is taking the calls, the patient might consider calling or visiting a 24-hour doctor service, outpatient clinic, or even an emergency room. Where there is a will, there is a way: you can always get more medication in almost any location. The patient's doctor can telephone a pharmacy or hospital even in a foreign country, or the patient can go to a local doctor or hospital. Bottom line: don't run out of medications!

Traveling Across Time Zones

Traveling across time zones poses two risks for breakthrough seizures: change in the person's day-wake (circadian) cycle that causes sleep deprivation and reduction in AED levels due to changing schedules. Shifting time zones can disrupt sleep. People with epilepsy should get plenty of sleep for the first 1–2 days after a greater than 1-hour shift in time zone. So if someone travels from New York to Paris, the first few days in Paris and the first few days after returning to New York, they should take it easy and get plenty of sleep.

When traveling across time zones, the amount of medication taken over a 24- or 48-hour period should remain constant, and the interval between doses should be approximately the same. Since changes in time zones increase the likelihood of sleep deprivation, better to err on the side of taking slightly too much medication or too-frequent doses than too little.

Each drug has a half-life—the time required for the drug's blood concentration to decline to half of its maximum value. Medications with a short half-life, such as gabapentin, pose a greater problem than those with a longer half-life, such as lamotrigine or zonisamide. For drugs with a short half-life, the interval between doses should be maintained as much as possible. Otherwise, side effects from high drug levels or seizures from low drug levels could result. It's not necessary to use an alarm clock to take the medications at exactly the same interval, however.

The timing with long half-life medications is less critical because the drug levels fluctuate less.

If the seizures have been difficult to control, if there are problems with dose-related side effects, or if time zone differences are confusing, the patient should ask the doctor about taking medications during travel. In some persons, benzodiazepines such as lorazepam (Ativan) or clonazepam (Klonopin) may increase sleep time on the plane, decrease jet lag, and reduce the risk of a seizure while traveling. Melatonin can be used to avoid jet lag (see below).

Sleep Deprivation

Sleep deprivation, or lack of restorative sleep, can trigger a seizure. Some people suffer a single seizure for the only time in their life after an "all-nighter" at college or during a prolonged period of poor sleep with a major life stress. Lack of proper sleep can increase their chances of a seizure or increase the intensity and duration of a seizure. Doctors take advantage of this phenomenon by asking persons with known or suspected epilepsy to stay up very late before an EEG to "activate the brain" and record abnormal epilepsy waves. Sleep deprivation also makes it more likely that the EEG will record sleep, increasing the chances of epilepsy waves in some people. Similarly, epilepsy centers use sleep deprivation during video-EEG recordings to help provoke a seizure.

We don't know why sleep deprivation provokes seizures. The sleep–wake cycle is associated with prominent changes in brain electrical, chemical, and hormonal activities. Seizures and the sleep–wake cycle are often related. Some people have all of their seizures in sleep or while awake, some have seizures transitioning into or out of sleep, and still others have seizures randomly spread throughout the day or night.

People with epilepsy should get adequate sleep—enough to feel refreshed the next day. In general, adults should try for at least 7–8 hours a night. Going to bed late (for example, 3 A.M. instead of 11 P.M.) can be compensated for by sleeping late (10 A.M. instead of 6 A.M.) and thereby avoiding sleep deprivation. However, for some, the disruption of the circadian rhythm may make seizures more likely even if they total sleep time is the same. Are you sleep-deprived? One good measure is the alarm clock—if you need one to wake up every morning, you are probably sleep deprived! Many people with epilepsy (and retired people) get into a different sleep rhythm, where they may sleep 4–5 hours at night but nap once or twice for an additional 2–4 hours during the day. Although they may feel as if they are not getting enough sleep, a log will often show that they are getting 7–8 hours per day.

For persons who have problems falling asleep and staying asleep, some simple measures can help: the sleeping environment should be quiet and dark, and they should avoid caffeinated beverages or foods within 6 hours of going to sleep, avoid alcohol, exercise daily but not within a few hours of going to sleep, and go to bed only when sleepy (not to read or watch TV).

Sleeping pills should be used only under a doctor's supervision and almost never for more than 2 or 3 weeks. During periods of tremendous stress, however, such as loss of a job or a relationship, the judicious use of sleeping pills for several nights can help to prevent a seizure caused by sleep deprivation. Even with short-term use, they must be handled carefully, because stopping certain types of sleeping pills, especially the benzodiazepines such as triazolam (Halcion), clonazepam (Klonopin), and temazepam (Restoril), can trigger seizures in susceptible persons. Other drugs also work at the benzodiazepine receptor but are not benzodiazepines, such as zolpiderm (Ambien), eszopiclone (Lunesta), and zaleplon (Sonesta). These drugs have less tendency to become habit-forming or cause seizures if suddenly discontinued after regular use. Ramelteon (Rozerem) targets melatonin receptors and has no potential to be habit-forming or cause withdrawal seizures; it is the only sleep medicine approved for long-term use. Melatonin is an over-the-counter drug that promotes sleep and can help regulate the sleep–wake cycle; it appears safe for most people with epilepsy. For sleep, 2–3 mg a half hour before bedtime is recommended. Diphenhydramine (Benadryl; also in over-the-counter sleep drugs such as Sominex) is not habit-forming, but, like other antihistamines, it can lower the seizure threshold and should generally be avoided by people with epilepsy.

Persons who become dependent on sleeping pills should consult their doctors about getting off of them. Gradual reduction of the dosage, possible substitution of non–habit-forming medications that promote sleep, and improved sleep hygiene can help.

Sleep disorders are common in the general population as well as in people with epilepsy. Sleep disorders include insomnia (trouble falling asleep, staying asleep, waking up too early), tiredness during the day, sleep apnea, and restless legs syndrome. Snoring can be a sign of sleep apnea. In children, snoring every night is abnormal. Sleep disorders impair restorative sleep and can therefore make seizures more likely to occur in both children and adults. If a sleep disorder is suspected, consider an evaluation by a sleep specialist.

Alcohol Use

Alcohol use can be followed by "withdrawal" seizures 4–72 hours after drinking has stopped. Alcohol in small to moderate amounts actually has properties to counteract seizures (antiepileptic effects), but it should never be consumed to control seizures. Withdrawal seizures are most common among persons who have abused alcohol for years. When alcohol consumption is stopped suddenly or markedly reduced over a short period of time, a seizure may occur. This is an example of provoked seizures rather than true epilepsy. In a similar way, the abrupt withdrawal of barbiturates or benzodiazepines can provoke seizures.

Long-standing alcohol abuse increases the risk of developing epilepsy. In such cases, multiple factors probably contribute, including repeated bouts of intoxication and withdrawal, head injury, and vitamin or mineral deficiencies.

Alcohol use by people with epilepsy is controversial. Alcohol withdrawal can also provoke seizures in a person with epilepsy. The risk of withdrawal seizures markedly increases after consuming three or more alcoholic drinks (1 drink = 5 oz. wine, 12 oz. beer, or 1.5 oz. of 80 proof liquor), but sensitive individuals may suffer withdrawal seizures after fewer drinks. Several studies found that adults with epilepsy may have one or two alcoholic beverages a day without any worsening of their seizures or changing AED levels.* A common problem is a young adult who drinks excessively, forgets his or her AEDs, and then suffers a withdrawal seizure.

---

*Acute consumption of three or more alcoholic beverages can inhibit metabolism of some AEDs (e.g., phenytoin) and lead to increased drug levels and an increased risk of side effects. Chronic use of alcohol will cause the liver enzymes that break down AEDs to work harder, resulting in lower drug levels and an increased risk of seizures.

People with epilepsy are less likely than others to use or abuse alcohol, largely due to doctors' restrictions and warnings with their medication. However, moderate to heavy alcohol consumption is never recommended for persons with epilepsy. Alcohol and some AEDs share similar adverse effects, such as tiredness, unsteadiness, and slurred speech. Combining alcohol and AEDs can be extremely dangerous when driving or using dangerous equipment.

Drug Abuse

Cocaine can cause seizures. All forms of cocaine consumption can cause seizures within seconds to hours. Seizures caused by cocaine are uniquely dangerous and may be associated with heart attacks, interruption of the heart's normal rhythm (cardiac arrhythmia), and death. Seizures caused by cocaine can occur in someone who has never had a seizure.

Amphetamines, like cocaine, are brain stimulants. They are prescribed to treat attention deficit disorder, hyperactivity, and narcolepsy. When used under a doctor'ssupervision, amphetamines and other stimulants appear to be safe for people with epilepsy unless they cause sleep deprivation. When amphetamines and related drugs are abused, however, they can lead to severe sleep deprivation, confusion, and psychiatric disorders and can increase the risk of seizures. Overdoses of amphetamines can cause severe tonic-clonic seizures, heart attacks, and death.

Marijuana (cannabis, pot) is obtained from the flowering tops of hemp plants. The active ingredient is tetrahydrocannabinol (THC). In the nineteenth century, marijuana was used to treat epilepsy. Animal studies suggest that THC and cannibidiol, another group of sunstances in marijuana, may have both antiepileptic as well as seizure-provoking effects. Some very preliminary studies in humans suggest that cannibidiol may reduce seizure frequency. Because benefits are unproven, it is illegal, and side effects occur, marijuana is not recommended to treat epilepsy. Further, as with alcohol, even if marijuana or one of its components had antiepileptic effects, abrupt withdrawal of the substance after recreational use could provoke seizures.

Nicotine (in tobacco) and *caffeine* (in coffee, tea, chocolate, and other foods) are drugs that are often used and abused in our society. There is no evidence that using nicotine or caffeine in usual amounts affects

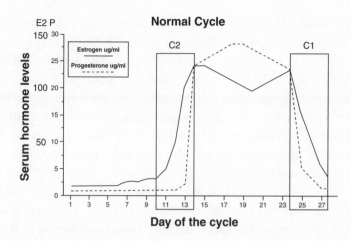

FIGURE 7.1: Hormonal changes during the menstrual cycle. Note that during ovulation (C2) and menstruation (C1), there is an increased ratio of estrogen (progesterone), making seizures more likely.

seizure control, but there are reports of susceptible persons in whom seizures were provoked by their abuse. Cigarette smoking also can be dangerous in persons who have seizures that impair consciousness or motor control, because a dropped cigarette can cause a fire.

Menstrual Cycle

Approximately one third of women of childbearing age with epilepsy report an increase in seizures around their monthly menstrual period, referred to as *catamenial epilepsy*. Seizures may occur shortly before menstruation, during and immediately after it, or at the time of ovulation (midcycle). The premenstrual and ovulatory phases are associated with the highest seizure frequencies (Fig. 7.1).

Hormonal changes are the most likely cause of increased seizures. The steroid sex hormones estrogen and progesterone alter the reactivity of brain nerve cells. In animals and humans, estrogen can cause or worsen seizures, whereas high doses of progesterone can act like an AED. High estrogen and/or low progesterone levels may be a critical factor in causing catamenial seizures.

Controlling catamenial seizures remains a difficult problem. For women who have regular menstrual cycles, a slight increase in the dosage of their usual AEDs or addition of acetazolamide (Diamox; a mild diuretic and AED) or benzodiazepine (such as lorazepam) just before and during the time of increased seizures may help. Neither birth control pills nor synthetic progesterone are effective. Menopause reduces the cyclic nature of the seizures, but is not associated with fewer seizures in most women with catamenial epilepsy. Natural progesterone may reduce catamenial seizures, but the effectiveness and safety remain to be established in controlled studies. One protocol uses progesterone lozenges (200 mg three times daily) on days 15–25 of each menstrual cycle, with gradual reduction over days 26–28. Side effects of progesterone include tiredness, breast tenderness, vaginal bleeding, and weight gain.

Stress

Stress affects brain function in many ways. Stress and the associated emotions of worry, fear, depression, frustration, and anger can cause sleep deprivation. Stress and anxiety can trigger an increase in the breathing rate (hyperventilation), which can provoke absence seizures. Stress and preoccupation with problems can cause some people to forget medication. Stress increases the steroid hormone cortisol, which may also influence seizure activity.

Stress may also directly affect brain areas and provoke seizures. The mechanism for this effect could involve the limbic system (deep parts of the temporal and frontal lobes), which regulates emotion. Seizures often arise from limbic aeras, so physiologic changes associated with intense or prolonged emotional states could increase seizure activity.

If seizures are more frequent with stress, try to avoid stressful situations and learn to minimize the impact of stress. The latter can be accomplished by exercise; relaxation techniques; yoga, tai chi, or other activities that involve both exercise and breathing techniques; as well as counseling or psychotherapy. However, none of us can completely avoid stress, and the worst stresses—the death of a loved one, serious injury, financial hardship—are often unpredictable. At these times, people with epilepsy should get enough sleep and not miss medications.

Stress is a frequently overlooked cause of seizures in children and people with mental handicaps. For both groups, it requires a balance of treating them like every other person who requires limits yet trying to minimize major stressors. For the mentally handicapped, stress can result from any change in their daily routine such as a new staff member at the residential home.

Over-the-Counter Drugs

Some over-the-counter drugs (bought without a doctor's prescription) can occasionally cause first-time seizures or provoke a seizure in a person with epilepsy (see Appendix C, page 357). Some cold, sleep, and allergy preparations contain diphenhydramine (Benadryl) and other antihistamines. Medications for runny and stuffed noses may contain pseudoephedrine or phenylephrine. These drugs have a small potential to cause seizures and should be avoided. In my experience, this is most important for those with primary generalized epilepsy. Diphenhydramine ointment applied to the skin for itching appears safe for people with epilepsy.

For aches, pains, and fevers, acetaminophen (e.g., Tylenol) and ibuprofen (e.g., Motrin, Advil) are the safest medications. Ibuprofen can increase blood levels of phenytoin and possibly cause side effects. Aspirin does not affect seizure threshold, but it should not be given to young children. Drug interactions may cause side effects if aspirin is taken by persons with high blood levels of valproate or phenytoin. Propoxyphene, another pain reliever in over-the-counter preparations, can increase blood carbamazepine levels and cause side effects.

Illness and Fever

Physical illness, from the respiratory flu to strep throat and appendicitis, may increase the risk that a person with epilepsy will have a seizure. Illness and fever are physical stressors, which, like emotional stressors, seem to have a nonspecific risk of making seizures more likely to occur. When people with epilepsy are ill, they should sleep well, avoid alcohol, and take prescribed medications. Gastrointestinal illnesses pose a special risk. Vomiting or diarrhea reduces the absorption of AEDs, which is especially dangerous in the setting of illness (see Chapter 11).

Nutritional Deficiencies

Many people are interested in pursuing dietary changes or taking nutritional supplements to improve seizure control. Foods can alter brain function, but reliable information is scarce. Very low levels of sugar in the blood (hypoglycemia) can cause seizures, especially in people with diabetes who take too much insulin or very rare patients with insulin-producing tumors. However, small reductions in blood sugar levels that often labeled as "hypoglycemia" have no known relationship to seizures or epilepsy. In general, people with epilepsy should eat a balanced diet. No nutritional supplement is known to improve seizure control except in rare cases of vitamin deficiencies (see Chapter 14).

Cycles of the Moon

The moon has been implicated in seizure occurrence for centuries. Modern neurology rarely considers the moon's cycles, but some adults and parents of children with epilepsy observe that seizures are more likely to occur during certain phases of the moon. The moon affects the magnetic and gravitational activities of the earth and can affect animal behavior. The relationship between the moon's phases and human behavior deserves study.

8 | The Health Care Team

Health care is a partnership. The notion that doctors give orders and patients follow them is old and unwise. People with epilepsy are part of the health care team; their input is critical for diagnosis and selecting and monitoring therapy. For example, the choice of AED may depend on the patient's feelings about side effects and expense. Many medical decisions are "judgment calls," which should reflect the shared knowledge and views of the patient and health professionals.

The Doctor and Patient

The doctor and patient are partners in health care; they share a common goal but have different responsibilities. For some patients, the doctor's visit is a passive event; the doctor checks them and makes recommendations. A visit should be interactive, however, because the doctor needs to know the patient's concerns and wishes. Some patients will do anything—even give up driving—to avoid taking medications. Others want to avoid seizures at almost any cost. These are very personal decisions. The treatment may need to change if a person's situation changes, such as a new job, marriage, or loss of health insurance.

Communication is central to a good patient–doctor relationship. The patient and family should provide accurate information. The doctor should use understandable language to discuss why tests are being obtained, what the tests involve, and the risks and benefits of therapy. Ideally, the relationship should be comfortable and based on trust. If you don't understand what the doctor says—tell them! If you have questions—ask them! Compared with past decades, doctors are now much more willing to share information and gain the patient's views about choices and potential risks.

Doctors in past generations benefited from more time with patients—time to listen, time to hear about the patient in their world. Today, patients may feel rushed, and their questions go unasked or unanswered. Busy doctors may appear more concerned about moving patients through the office, ordering tests, and prescribing drugs than hearing about the patient's life and problems. Make the visit with your doctor as productive as possible by focusing on your health and how it impacts your life.

The First Visit

You can foster a more productive interaction with the doctor. The doctor often begins by asking about the main problem and may then ask the patient to give a detailed account of the symptoms and their course over time. The doctor may question the patient carefully about events surrounding the seizure: Could it have been provoked by sleep deprivation, excessive use of alcohol, or some other factor? What was the setting? Did the episode occur shortly after standing? Was there a warning? Exactly what happened during the episode? How long did it last? Was the patient tired or confused after the episode? When did the patient first seek medical attention? What tests were done? What medication was prescribed? What was the response to the medication? Have there been more episodes? What were they like?

Try to prepare a brief written summary of the medical history. Although the referring doctor may write a letter summarizing the history, a summary by the patient or family is still helpful. Bring as many relevant medical records as possible, such as notes from other doctors, seizure calendars (records of seizures), and results of laboratory studies such as drug levels, EEG, and MRI reports. The actual MRI films or CD and EEG printouts or CD can be copied or borrowed.

Patients often find it helpful to bring a written list of questions, particularly if the purpose of the visit is to define issues or obtain specific answers. Questions are best asked at the end of the visit, after the doctor has heard the history, reviewed laboratory studies, and performed the examination. Try to limit the list to five questions; others can be saved for a future visit. In some doctor's offices and clinics, a nurse reviews the doctor's information and recommendations. The nurse can answer many questions and provide reading materials. This is often helpful, especially if the patient did not understand some of the doctor's comments.

When patients leave the doctor's office, they should understand the treatment plan and it should make sense. If not, or if important issues remain unresolved, ask more questions. Ask for written instructions, particularly on how to take medications. Know what to do if another seizure occurs or if medication is missed. If questions come up after leaving the doctor's office, call back and ask. Many questions can be answered by the nurse. Less important questions or bits of information— e.g., an uncle has epilepsy—can be communicated by a note or at the next visit.

Follow-Up Visits

Follow-up doctor's appointments usually last 10–30 minutes. If the patient is seizure-free and tolerating the medications, the visit may be brief. If the seizures are worse or the medications have caused new side effects, the visit often needs to be longer. If there is a need to discuss special subjects, such as pregnancy, discontinuing AEDs, or epilepsy surgery, a longer appointment may be required. Let the doctor's office know if additional time is needed (there may be some additional charge).

There is often a gap between the doctor's perception of how the patient is doing and how the patient feels he or she is doing. Doctors may have no idea about how the patient experiences his or her disorder. For example, some patients are most fearful of a seizure causing embarrassment, others injury, and others side effects of medication. Often, if things are "stable," the doctor may assume they are "ok" when they are not. Let the doctor know how epilepsy affects you and your family—it can help them better care for you. Balancing seizure control and side effects is a science and an art that varies by doctor, patient, and AED(s). In some cases, medication doses that provide complete seizure freedom may produce disabling side effects. Reducing or changing the AED to alleviate these effects may come at the cost of some seizure activity, but may provide a better overall balance. For example, 2 minutes of mild seizure activity per month and minimal side effects may be better for some people than seizure freedom with tiredness and dizziness most of every day.

Never adjust AEDs without consulting the doctor. If a drug is unaffordable or the medication is causing problems, tell your doctor. Although discussions about sensitive issues such as sexual desire or function, mood, or strange and embarrassing thoughts may feel uncomfortable, these should be discussed if they are a problem. If the doctor does not respond, make sure he or she understands how seriously the problem affects you or your loved one; speak to the nurse if possible. If repeated efforts to make the doctor aware of the problem are unsuccessful, consider changing doctors.

Financial Issues and Insurance Coverage

Most doctors have office or business managers who can answer questions about financial concerns or insurance coverage. In cases of financial hardship, many doctors are willing to accept payment plans or reduced fees. Managed care and health maintenance organizations vary in their coverage and access to specialty care, such as care by an epileptologist (an epilepsy specialist). Although many patients are well cared for by general neurologists, epileptologists are often more knowledgeable about new AEDs or issues such as pregnancy or possible surgical therapy. Lists of epileptologists can be obtained from websites (epilepsy.com, epilepsyfoundation.org). Epilepsy Foundation (EF) affiliates may know of doctors who accept certain insurances, reduced rates, or free clinics.

Patients with Medicaid can often obtain good care at public clinics in teaching hospitals. Teaching hospitals often have an epilepsy clinic supervised by an epileptologist, although residents or fellows in training may directly provide the care. The residents' and fellows' fund of knowledge and experience varies tremendously. They should be supervised by a senior doctor, and the patient should try to speak with the attending doctor. Since residents often change assignments, the attending doctor can provide more continuity of care.

Medicare reimburses doctors more fairly than Medicaid does, and most doctors accept Medicare (see Chapter 31). Medicare allows physicians to charge certain maximum rates for services. These rates are often lower than the standard rates charged for a service to a person who does not have Medicare.

Worker's compensation programs are regulated by the state and have fixed fees for medical services. Many doctors do not accept this coverage.

Second Opinions and Changing Doctors

If the doctor is not meeting a patient's needs, it may be worth obtaining a second opinion or changing doctors. Before doing this, however, the patient should consider again the areas in which he or she feels uncertain. In many cases, the patient may begin to feel more comfortable after asking the doctor additional questions or raising certain issues. When a second opinion is obtained, the patient often finds that the first doctor left no stone unturned and the second doctor agrees with all aspects of the care. However, the second doctor may have helpful suggestions regarding tests or changes in therapy.

Many patients are initially cared for by a primary care doctor (general practitioner, internist, or pediatrician). A neurologist should always be consulted. If after having been treated by a neurologist for 6–12 months seizures remain uncontrolled or AED side effects are troublesome, the patient should be referred to an epileptologist.

For a second opinion, either ask the current doctor for an epileptologist or obtain a name from a reliable source (see above), or another patient. Care should be coordinated. The first doctor should communicate with and send the patient's records to the epileptologist. The patient usually continues care with the first doctor, but should be comfortable switching if he or she so chooses.

Changing doctors may be awkward and uncomfortable. In some cases, communication and trust between the patient and the doctor may break down. Problems can arise, for example, over time spent during the visit, promptness in returning phone calls, finances, AED side effects, failure to take medication as prescribed, or language difficulties. Relationships have chemistry, and the chemistry may not be right. The patient should call the doctor's office and tell them that he or she is changing doctors. Write a brief note asking that the records be forwarded to the new doctor or directly to the patient (so you can make and keep a copy). Patients have a legal right to their medical records. The note can be very simple: "Please forward all of my medical records to Dr. —," and give the doctor's address. Call the new doctor's office before the appointment to make sure that the records have arrived. There may be a charge for copying the records, but there are limits on these charges.

Patients should avoid burning bridges behind them when changing doctors. There may be only two neurologists or epileptologists in a community, and the patient may turn out to like the original one better than the second one, for example, or the original neurologist may be on-call when the patient is brought in for an emergency room visit.

The Nurse

Nurses are on the front line of medicine. In the emergency room, they often first obtain clinical information. In the clinic, they often participate in the patient's visit and help fully explain the test or describe exactly how to take the drugs. Nurses often translate the doctor's explanations and instructions into a more comprehensible language and less intimidating setting and provide written instructions and educational material. In many medical offices, nurses answer questions over the phone and in person. The nurse may spend more time with the patient than the doctor. Patients should feel comfortable talking with the nurse about problems and should have confidence in the nurse's response. If patients want to speak with the doctor, however, or want the nurse to check with the doctor, they should ask.

The Nurse-Clinician

Nurse-clinicians are specially trained to help assess, coordinate, and implement patient education and care. They can answer routine questions over the phone, such as those about laboratory results, upcoming tests, adverse effects of medications, dosage schedules, interactions between AEDs and other medications, and the safety of activities. Nurse-clinicians can also make referrals to another doctor, a social worker, or a therapist.

The Nurse Practitioner

Nurse practitioners are nurses with advanced medical education. They are licensed to take a medical history, examine patients, order tests, and prescribe medications, including narcotics and other restricted substances. Nurse practitioners serve as relatively independent practitioners who diagnose and treat patients. They are supervised by doctors, who review case histories and treatment plans at regular intervals.

The Physician Assistant

Physician assistants help doctors in obtaining the medical history, examining the patient, recommending therapy, drawing blood, ordering tests, speaking with consulting doctors, and many other functions. In most states, physician assistants can prescribe medications.

The Social Worker-Counselor

Social workers are often invaluable members of the epilepsy care team, but those with expertise in epilepsy may only be found in epilepsy centers. Social workers play many roles, from educating the patient or family or community members about epilepsy to assisting in identifying and obtaining precious resources, including:

- Special education programs
- Respite centers (where a child or adult with special needs can spend time to give caregivers a rest)
- Home health aides
- Medical insurance benefits

- ✒ Vocational rehabilitation centers

- ✒ Referrals to psychologists and other mental health workers

- ✒ Referrals to fight discrimination; advocacy groups (local Protection and Advocacy Service, Legal Aid Society), or an attorney specializing in this subject

Social workers are often invaluable members of the epilepsy care team, especially inepilepsy centers. The counseling sessions provide a place to discuss social and personal issues that may not be addressed elsewhere. Counseling sessions are also beneficial for children, helping them to understand issues of independence, maturity, and personal growth.

The EEG Technologist

The EEG is a recording of the electrical activity of the brain (see Chapter 9). The EEG technologist performs the EEG test. He or she explains the testing procedure to the patient, obtains some background information (age, diagnosis, medications, time of last meal, time of last seizure), and then applies the electrodes to the patient's scalp, records the EEG, and prepares the EEG record for the doctor's review. The director of the EEG laboratory supervises the EEG technologist.

The EEG session takes about an hour, allowing the technologist to learn about the patient's life and their epilepsy. This information can help the health care team.

The Pharmacist

Pharmacists fill prescriptions and dispense drugs. But they also help discuss the potential side effects and interactions of medications with each other and over-the-counter, herbal, and other products. Pharmacists also monitor the costs of drugs and, together with your doctor, can help assess relative risks and cost benefits of generic versus brand-name drugs (see Chapter 11).

Many people feel more comfortable talking to their pharmacist than to their doctor. Pharmacists are knowledgeable and can provide expert information about medications, but they cannot substitute for doctors.

Epilepsy Associations and Support Groups

The Epilepsy Foundation local affiliates (see Chapter 33) and community or epilepsy-center–based support groups are important resources. These groups are sometimes directed by a social worker or counselor. Depending on the specific group, services include support group meetings to discuss social and related issues, lectures on health issues, referrals for vocational rehabilitation, lectures to schoolchildren and school nurses about epilepsy, and assistance with medical and other referrals.

Specialty Members of the Health Care Team

The health care team is defined by the needs of the patient. In epilepsy centers, consultation with a neuropsychologist and psychiatrist is common, especially when surgery is considered. Specialists in vocational rehabilitation, physical therapy, occupational therapy, music therapy, speech therapy, or special education are important for selected patients.

The Neuropsychologist

Neuropsychologists assess intellectual and behavioral function. The neuropsychologist or an assistant administers tests that help to identify relative strengths and weaknesses in areas such as thinking, reasoning, memory, language, perception, motor ability, and behavior. For example, memory, a problem for many people with epilepsy, can be carefully studied. These tests are essential in the assessment for epilepsy surgery, but they can also monitor changes in certain intellectual functions.

The neuropsychologist can help define the cognitive effects of a brain injury from head trauma, stroke, or tumor. For example, frontal lobe injury from trauma may affect judgment and motivation, making it difficult to understand why regular medication use and avoiding excessive alcohol use are important. Neuropsychologists also perform therapy or other interventions for intellectual or behavioral problems and private psychotherapy for emotional problems related to brain disorders.

For patients considering epilepsy surgery, the neuropsychologist often helps perform the intracarotid sodium amobarbital test (see Chapter 13) and electrical stimulation of the brain to map areas of intellectual functions, such as speech.

The Psychiatrist

Many of psychological and psychiatric problems (e.g., depression, anxiety, and psychosis) are more common in people with epilepsy than the general population and can occur in approximately half of those with poorly controlled seizures. Although people often have negative feelings about psychiatrists, mainly because of stigmas associated with behavioral disorders and misconceptions about psychiatric care, they are often essential.

Depression is a common problem among people with epilepsy. It may be caused by medications, psychosocial problems (loss of a job, problems from epilepsy), and biological factors such as brain injuries (e.g., trauma) and epilepsy. The biological processes that underlie epilepsy may predispose toward depression and other behavioral disorders. The psychiatrist can diagnose the problem, determine its cause, and recommend treatment, such as adjusting AEDs, adding an antidepressant drug, or counseling the patient.

Chemistry is often an essential part of the psychiatrist-patient relationship. If the patient has a behavioral problem and is not comfortable with a particular psychiatrist, he or she should consider seeing another doctor rather than concluding that "psychiatry failed." Communication between the psychiatrist and epilepsy doctor helps coordinate care.

The Psychologist

Psychologists can help people understand and cope with epilepsy as a neurological disorder and as a social stigma. They can guide patients and their families in learning to live more positively and productively. Their counseling role is similar to social workers, and they can help treat mood disorders and problems with self-esteem and independence. As someone to talk to about life stresses and the influences of epilepsy, its treatment, and its consequences, psychologists can be a much-needed resource. Psychologists can provide cognitive-behavioral therapy, a form of psychotherapy that focuses on changing thought patterns to change how people feel and act.

The Physical Therapist

Physical therapists help people who have disorders of movement, coordination, or sensation to become more physically able. Mobility and coordination can be enhanced through stretching, exercise, and skills development. Individuals with limited mobility or other physical disorders can benefit.

The Occupational Therapist

Occupational therapists help individuals with disorders that affect their ability to perform daily tasks, especially ones requiring fine motor control, such as writing.

The Speech-Language Pathologist

Speech-language pathologists assist people with speech, language, and swallowing disorders. Speech therapists assess the nature of the problem and recommend a program of therapy, which varies depending on the problems and the approach of the specific therapist.

The Vocational Rehabilitation Counselor

Vocational rehabilitation counselors help people with disabilities to obtain skills needed for employment. Specialized programs, some of which are sponsored by state or community agencies, may be available to facilitate this process (see Chapter 33). Counselors can help by assessing knowledge, skills, and interests and recommending areas to pursue. They teach people how to accommodate and overcome aspects of their disability, improve work habits, train for specific job functions, develop better interviewing skills, and seek and obtain employment.

One young man who was seizure-free after epilepsy surgery had difficulty obtaining a job in the printing industry, where he had worked for more than 7 years. After a brief vocational rehabilitation program trained him with computers, he found a job and was promoted twice in the year.

The Comprehensive Epilepsy Center

Epilepsy centers (see Chapter 33) are valuable resources for any person with definite or suspected epilepsy who has unresolved problems related to the disorder. Patients may be referred to a comprehensive epilepsy center for a single outpatient visit for an assessment of their current diagnosis and therapy, or they may receive longer-term care.

9 | Making the Diagnosis of Epilepsy

T he diagnosis of epilepsy is usually straightforward, but it can be difficult since many other disorders cause sudden behavioral changes that are similar to seizure symptoms. The correct diagnosis depends on an accurate description of the events occurring before, during, and after the attack. The patient and witness of the event should give the doctor as much information as possible. If certain details are vague, the doctor should be told. No matter how accurate and complete the information, however, some episodes remain difficult even for experts to diagnose. Every epilepsy specialist has had patients for whom their initial diagnosis was incorrect. This is one reason that follow-up care, and the additional information it provides, is essential. Also, some patients have more than one type of seizure.

Conditions Confused with Epilepsy

Many medical, neurological, and psychiatric disorders can mimic seizures. The correct therapy depends on the correct diagnosis. Only a few disorders that are most often mistaken for an epileptic seizure are

presented here. Chapter 24 discusses some conditions occurring only in
children that can be confused with seizures.

Fainting

Sara came to the Epilepsy Center because she had five
episodes of dizziness followed by loss of consciousness over
6 months. Witnesses said her arms jerked and her eyes had
"rolled up in her head"; people said they were seizures. The
neurologist found that all the events happened when she
was dehydrated or after experiencing pain. Sara underwent a
prolonged EEG study that was normal and had a tilt table test
that showed that her blood pressure dropped abnormally in
certain positions. Sara was reassured by her neurologist that
she had neurogenic syncope—a fancy word for fainting—not
epileptic seizures.

Fainting (syncope) occurs when the brain does not receive enough
blood, oxygen, or sugar. Fainting, a brief loss of consciousness, is common
and rarely serious. Most often the person is standing and complains of
some combination of dizziness, lightheadedness, abdominal discomfort,
and blurry vision, turns pale, sweats, and then falls. The body may stiffen
slightly, and the arms or legs may jerk several times. The misdiagnosis of
an epileptic seizure may be made when the doctor hears that someone
suddenly lost consciousness, fell down, and had jerking movements. In
rare cases, a faint can evolve into a full-blown convulsive seizure. In most
cases of fainting, consciousness is lost for less than 1 minute, and the
person is alert 10–30 seconds later. Falling is a natural remedy for the
faint. Many faints result from the heart's inability to pump blood up to
the brain, so when the person is horizontal, blood flows more easily
to the head.

Many disorders can cause fainting. A common cause is orthostatic
hypotension—a drop in blood pressure when someone arises from a
lying or sitting position. Common contributing causes include dehydration from inadequate fluid intake, increased sweating, diarrhea, or
vomiting, as well as prolonged standing in a hot environment. Fainting

may result froma disturbance in the rhythm of the heart (e.g., prolonged QT syndrome, ventricular tachycardia, or fibrillation), which often requires treatment.

Hypoglycemia

Hypoglycemia (low blood sugar) is overdiagnosed. It is a serious medical problem in some people, most often diabetics who take too much insulin. An endocrine tumor of the pancreas is an extremely rare cause. Hypoglycemia can cause dizziness, lightheadedness, fainting, and convulsive seizures.

Unfortunately, hypoglycemia is often diagnosed without good evidence. The diagnosis of hypoglycemia is often based on the results of a glucose tolerance test, in which a high sugar content drink is given and changes in blood sugar (glucose) are measured over the next several hours. Low blood sugar levels on this test commonly occur in perfectly healthy individuals. The diagnosis of hypoglycemia is supported by low blood sugar levels when symptoms are present and consuming sugar or other carbohydrates leads to a resolution of symptoms.

Sleep Attacks

In sleep attacks, a person has an irresistible urge to sleep and suddenly dozes off, usually for only minutes. Upon awakening, he or she feels refreshed. Sleep attacks may be a symptom of narcolepsy, a sleep disorder. These attacks usually occur during boring conditions, but can occur in dangerous settings such as driving. People with narcolepsy may also suffer sudden loss of muscle tone, causing them to, for example, drop things, nod their head, or fall, when they experience strong emotions such as vigorous laughing or crying.

Sleep Apnea

Sleep apnea is a condition in which breathing is intermittently (often frequently) interrupted during sleep. Most patients snore loudly. Their sleep is restless with frequent brief awakenings. The disrupted sleep can cause excessive daytime sleepiness, irritability, and impaired thinking. In someone with epilepsy, sleep apnea can worsen seizure control by impairing restful sleep.

Nonepileptic (Psychogenic) Seizures

> Despite the use of many seizure medications, Jennifer, a 30-year-old woman, had frequent episodes of shaking and impaired responsiveness that did not stop with emergency medications. An epilepsy specialist recorded several of her episodes on video EEG and diagnosed nonepileptic seizures. After months of working closely with her neurologist, neuro-psychiatrist, and psychologist, Jennifer has had no more episodes. She is off all medications and has resumed driving.

Nonepileptic (psychogenic) seizures are attacks that resemble epileptic seizures but result from subconscious mental activity, not abnormal brain electrical activity. Doctors consider most of these episodes psychological in nature, but not purposely produced. The person is usually unaware that the attacks are not "epileptic." Non epileptic seizures are common, and patients may be incorrectly treated for epileptic seizures for decades until the correct diagnosis is made. Nonepileptic seizures are most common in adolescents and adults but also can occur in children and the elderly. They are three times more common in women. Approximately 20% of patients with these seizures also have epileptic seizures and require different treatment for each disorder.

Nonepileptic seizures most often imitate complex partial or tonic-clonic seizures. The degree of resemblance varies considerably. Because doctors rarely witness an attack, the diagnosis is often delayed. Family members report episodes in which the patient stares or stiffens and jerks, and doctors misdiagnose epilepsy. Certain features suggest nonepileptic seizures:

- Wild movements such as thrashing or rolling from side to side
- Screaming, crying, and moaning
- Jerking or stiffening of all extremities but with preserved consciousness
- Stiffening and jerking of the extremities with immediate resumption of normal alertness after the attack (tiredness or confusion typically occurs after a tonic-clonic seizure)

> Altered behavior that waxes and wanes (jerking or the inability to respond to questions comes and goes)

> Prolonged episodes, lasting longer than 5 minutes

No single feature is diagnostic. Epileptic seizures may occasionally include one or more of these behaviors.

Nonepileptic seizures are usually diagnosed with video-EEG monitoring; approximately 20% of patients referred to epilepsy centers for video-EEG have nonepileptic seizures. Doctors often try to have a family member or friend observe the recorded attack to ensure that it is similar to the usual episodes. Suggestive techniques help provoke a nonepileptic seizure.

The treatment of nonepileptic seizures varies with the underlying psychological issues. Sometimes, when the doctor tells the person that the attacks are psychological, they stop. Coexisting depression or anxiety disorders may require medication. The prognosis for resolution of the disorder and for the patient's psychological well-being varies. Counseling or psychotherapy is often helpful. Accepting the diagnosis (at least as a real possibility) and following through with therapy are essential for a successful outcome.

Panic Attacks

Panic attacks are episodes of profound fear and anxiety, often associated with increased heart and breathing rate, shortness of breath, sweating, nausea, chest discomfort, and other bodily (autonomic) symptoms. Certain settings may precipitate panic attacks. Doctors may incorrectly suspect that the person is suffering from partial seizures, because simple partial seizures may have both autonomic and emotional symptoms such as fear or anxiety. Unlike seizures, which begin suddenly and usually last less than 3 minutes, panic attacks often build up gradually and last longer than 5 minutes. Many individuals with panic attacks also suffer from depression, and antidepressant medications can treat both disorders.

The Medical History

The medical history is the foundation for diagnosing epilepsy. The doctor should be given all information about the seizure, because most doctors never witness a patient's actual attack. The following questions may be asked:

Before the attack:

⚬ Was there lack of sleep or unusual stress?

⚬ Was there any recent illness?

⚬ Had the person taken any medications or drugs, including over-the-counter drugs, alcohol, or illegal drugs?

⚬ What was the person doing immediately before the attack: lying, sitting, standing, getting up from a lying position, heavy exercise?

During the attack:

⚬ What time of day did it occur?

⚬ Did it occur around the transition into or out of sleep?

⚬ How did it begin?

⚬ Was there a warning?

⚬ Were there abnormal movements of the eyes, mouth, face, head, arms, or legs?

⚬ Was the person able to talk and respond appropriately?

⚬ Was there loss of urine or feces?

⚬ Was the tongue or inside of the cheeks bitten?

After the attack:

⚬ Was the person confused or tired?

⚬ Was speech normal?

⚬ Was there a headache?

⚬ Was any part of the body weak?

An accurate description of the typical attack from an eyewitness is invaluable. Ask the witnesses to write down a detailed description since memories fade, and if possible, come to the doctor's office, or speak with the doctor or nurse about their observations. Save these witnesses' notes, as they can help another doctor. If the episodes recur, try to capture them on home video.

Patients should review their past history with family members. Was their birth difficult or traumatic? Were there seizures with fever in infancy or early childhood? Was there a head injury with loss of consciousness? If yes, how long was consciousness lost and were they taken to a hospital? Did they ever have meningitis (infection of the membranes around the brain and spinal cord) or encephalitis (viral infection of the brain)? Has anyone else in the family had epilepsy or any other neurological disorder, or a disorder associated with loss of consciousness or symptoms similar to those of the patient?

If the episodes recur, try to identify associated factors. For example, some women have more frequent seizures around menstruation. Although it is tempting to link seizures with specific environmental factors (e.g., antibiotic use, increased sugar or NutraSweet consumption, stress) these associations are often coincidental. Careful documentation of when the possible factor occurs in relation to seizures can help establish an association, but a relationship does not prove causatian.

The General Medical Examination

Because seizures may result from medical disorders, a general medical examination is part of the first consultation. An examination and laboratory studies can assess the functioning of the liver, kidneys, and other organ systems. The neurologist should know about medical disorders such as hyperthyroidism or kidney disease. The primary doctor may have insights into illnesses that cause or contribute to seizures. If an AED is recommended, the interactions with medications taken for a medical disorder must be considered.

The Neurological Examination

Identifying whether there is an area of abnormal brain function is the essence of the neurological examination. The neurologist assesses mental functions, such as the ability to remember words, calculate, and name objects, and will then systematically test the functioning of the muscles and senses, along with reflexes, walking, and coordination.

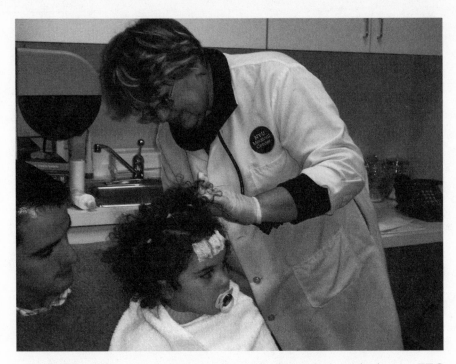

FIGURE 9.1: A patient being set up with electrodes attached to an EEG machine.

A brief screening examination is often done during follow-up visits to identify any changes in neurological function. If the patient has slurred speech, impaired concentration, difficulty walking a straight line with heels touching the toes, jerking eye movements when the eyes are directed toward one side, or trembling when the arms are outstretched, the AED dosage may need to be reduced. Follow-up exams are usually brief, especially if there are no new complaints. Therefore, the doctor's time is often better spent listening than examining, although the neurologist examines while listening (e.g., mood, thinking, language, eye and facial movements, etc.).

The EEG

Electroencephalography is the most specific test for diagnosing epilepsy, because it records the brain's electrical activity. It is a safe and painless procedure in which electrodes are applied to the patient's scalp (Fig. 9.1)

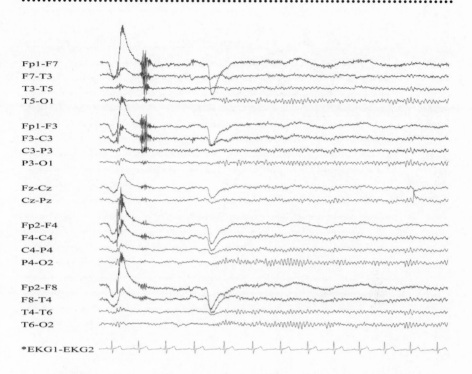

FIGURE 9.2: EEG traces from a person without epilepsy, at rest. Each line corresponds to an area of the brain from which the EEG recording was made.

and connected by wires to an electrical box, which in turn is connected to an EEG machine. The EEG technologist first measures the patient's head so that the electrodes, which are small, metal, cup-shaped disks attached to wires, can be placed in the correct position. A wax crayon, which can be easily washed off later, may mark the points on the scalp. Next, the technologist applies the electrodes, usually using a paste that holds them in place. The technologist may gently scrub each position with a mildly abrasive cream before applying the electrodes to improve the quality of the recording. The EEG digitally records the brain waves as a series of squiggly lines (older machines use paper). The EEG does not stimulate the head with electricity and poses no danger.

The EEG machine records the brain's electrical activity as a series of squiggles called traces (Fig. 9.2). Each trace corresponds to a different region of the brain. The wires can only record electrical activity; they do not deliver electrical current.

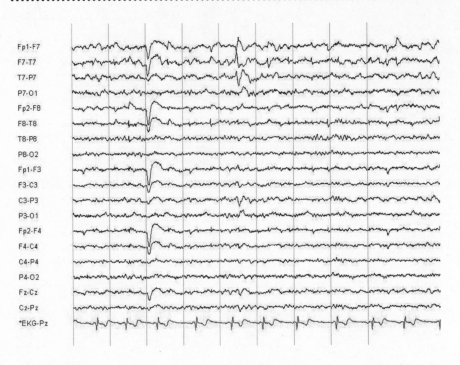

FIGURE 9.3: EEG traces of spikes and sharp waves (epilepsy waves) from the left temporal lobe of a person with partial epilepsy. The four traces on the bottom, which are from the right frontal and temporal lobes, are normal.

The EEG shows well-defined patterns of normal or abnormal brain electrical activity. Abnormal patterns may be either nonspecific or specific. Nonspecific patterns are seen in many different conditions. For example, slow waves can occur after head trauma, stroke, brain tumor, migraine, or seizures. Slow waves have a lower frequency (cycles per second) than expected for the patient's age. Epilepsy waves (spikes, sharp waves, and spike-and-wave discharges) are specific patterns that indicate a tendency toward seizures. Spikes and sharp waves occurring in a local area of the brain, such as the left temporal lobe, are seen in patients with partial epilepsy (Fig. 9.3). Spike-and-wave discharges beginning simultaneously over both hemispheres are markers of primary generalized epilepsy (Fig. 9.4). In some cases, seizures are recorded during the EEG, particularly in children with absence seizures during increased breathing (hyperventilation).

Because the EEG usually records the brain activity between seizures, which is called interictal activity (ictal means seizure-related), a person

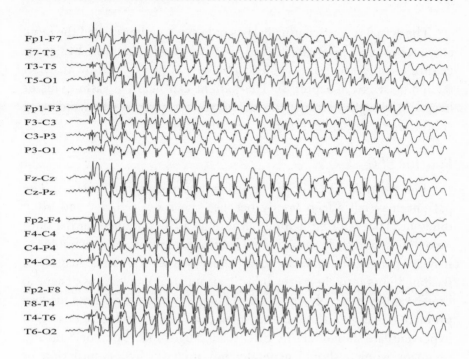

FIGURE 9.4: EEG traces of spike-and-wave discharges from both the left and right sides of the brain in a person with primary generalized epilepsy.

with epilepsy may have a normal EEG during a random 30-minute sampling. Just as seizures occupy a tiny percentage of a patient's life, the EEG can be normal for many epilepsy patients. Also, areas of abnormality may go undetected by the EEG if the activity arises from deep regions "outside the reach" of the scalp electrodes, or if the volume of brain affected is too small to generate abnormal waves of sufficient size. To increase the chances of finding an abnormality on the EEG, it can be recorded in various circumstances:

- During both wakefulness and sleep
- After sleep deprivation
- With 3–5 minutes of deep breathing (hyperventilation)
- With flashing lights (photic stimulation)
- With special electrodes
- For prolonged periods

The actual recording usually lasts only 20–40 minutes, and the same amount of time is generally needed to prepare for it. Thus, the EEG procedure usually takes 1–1½ hours. The test is performed by an EEG technologist (see Chapter 8). The patient can help by washing his or her hair the night before or the day of the test, but should avoid using conditioners, hair creams, sprays, or styling gels.

Routine EEG

The routine EEG is the most common test for epilepsy. The patient may fall asleep briefly because the room is quiet and often dimly lit. That is often helpful because an EEG obtained during both wakefulness and sleep may provide extra information. The technologist may ask patients to open and close their eyes several times, may shine flashing lights into their eyes (photic stimulation), or may ask them to breath rapidly or deeply (hyperventilation). Patients who have a medical problem, such as asthma or heart disease, which makes it unsafe to hyperventilate should tell the EEG technologist or the doctor. Similarly, pregnant women should generally not undergo hyperventilation or photic stimulation. The doctor may ask the patient to be sleep deprived before the EEG to increase the chance of recording epilepsy waves. If any possible seizure symptoms occur during the test, the patient should tell the technologist.

Obtaining an EEG in children is usually easy, but it can be challenging. For babies, it is helpful to perform the EEG around naptime. Electrodes can be applied while the mother holds the child; a bottle may help to calm the baby. Then the baby can sleep naturally. Some babies and young children require sedation to apply the electrodes and record sleep activity.

After the EEG is done, the technologist removes the electrodes and much of the paste. The paste is lanolin- or water-based, so the rest can be easily washed off at home. The doctor usually reads the EEG after patient has left.

EEG with Special Electrodes

Depending on the information the doctor is trying to obtain, special electrodes may be needed. Sphenoidal electrodes (see Chapter 13) may be used during video-EEG monitoring studies to record electrical activity from deep parts of the temporal and frontal lobes. The patient's cheek is swabbed with an anesthetic to minimize pain, and then a thin needle, which carries a thin wire, is inserted into the cheek. The needle is removed, and the wire is taped to the skin. Patients usually experience little discomfort.

Ambulatory EEG

The brain's electrical activity fluctuates from second to second. The routine 20- to 40-minute EEG is often too short to capture epilepsy waves or seizures. An extended recording with long periods of wakefulness and sleep is desired.

A special recorder, slightly larger than a portable cassette player, can capture 24–72 hours of EEG while the patients can go about most of their usual activities. Video recording capacity may also be available. Epilepsy wave and seizure detection programs help identify abnormal activity. The recorder fits in a small carrying case, with the wires running either under or outside of their shirt (Fig. 9.5). Most people prefer not to go to work or school. Because the electrodes must stay on the head for a longer time than for a routine EEG, a special glue called collodion is often used. The technologist can remove this glue with acetone or similar solutions, although the last bit can be hard to get out.

If the patient scratches his or her head, which may get itchy because of the electrodes, it can appear as abnormal activity on the EEG. Therefore, patients should keep a diary of activities. Most recorders have an "event" button for patients or family members to press if typical seizure symptoms occur, such as episodes of feeling "spacey" or confused.

Video-EEG Monitoring

Video-EEG monitoring has revolutionized the diagnosis of epilepsy. It allows prolonged recording of the patient's behavior (audio and video) and the EEG, which can be viewed on a split screen. This permits a precise correlation of brain electrical activity and behavior during episodes (Fig. 9.6). Video-EEG recordings can be done on hospitalized inpatients or on outpatients. During video-EEG recordings, electrodes are usually glued to the scalp with collodion.

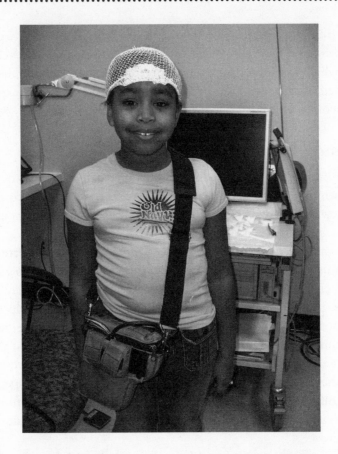

FIGURE 9.5: Recording the 24-hour ambulatory EEG. The device records the EEG signals from the electrodes on the patient's scalp while she pursues her daily activities.

Inpatient monitoring with close supervision allows the doctor to reduce or discontinue AEDs safely. Medication reduction, sleep deprivation, hyperventilation, exercise, or alcohol intake may be used to induce seizures. Video-EEG can help determine whether episodes are epileptic seizures and, if so, the type of seizures and the region of the brain from which the seizures begin. This last step is critical to evaluate if surgery is possible.

A patient who is going to have video-EEG monitoring should bring clothing to the hospital that can be buttoned, not pullovers. The patient should also bring reading materials and things to keep busy, as a hospital stay can be boring.

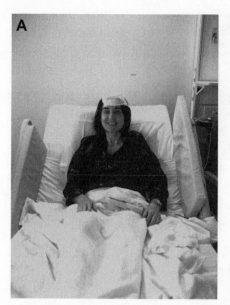
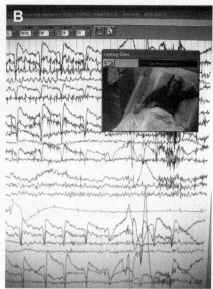

FIGURE 9.6: Video-EEG monitoring. **(A)** A patient being monitored; a video camera (not shown) records her activities, including any seizures that occur, and the EEG signals from electrodes on her head are transmitted to an adjoining monitor. **(B)** The patient's seizure and EEG are recorded simultaneously and shown as a split-screen display on a television monitor.

Magnetoencephalography (MEG)

MEG records the brain's magnetic activity. Because the physical properties of magnetic waves differ from those of electrical waves, MEG provides information that is complementary to the EEG. The EEG and MEG are usually recorded simultaneously to compare the activities. MEG uses detectors near the head (Fig. 9.7) that are painless and safe. The magnetic waves recorded between seizures can be three-dimensionally mapped onto an MRI image (Fig. 9.7B). The equipment used to record and analyze the MEG information is complex and costly, making the procedure expensive. MEG is available at a limited number of medical centers, and although it is approved by Medicare and supported by a large quantity of literature, some insurance companies do not cover the test or require letters of medical necessity and appeals to approve it.

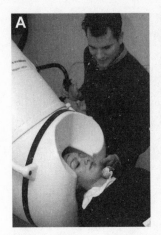
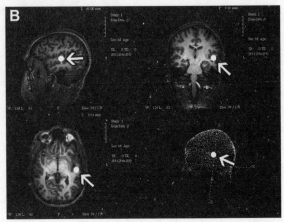

FIGURE 9.7: (A) A magnetoencephalograph (MEG) machine. **(B)** MEG area of epilepsy wave mapped onto an MRI image.

MEG's main use is to localize the area from which the seizure arises in patients undergoing evaluation for epilepsy surgery and to pinpoint the sites of normal sensory function (e.g., touch, vision) so that these vital areas can be spared. MEG is especially helpful in potential surgical cases when the seizures arise near functional tissue, outside the temporal lobe, and in patients with Landau-Kleffner syndrome.

Neuroimaging of the Brain

Neuroimaging provides pictures of the brain. The neuroimaging tests most commonly used with epilepsy are CT and MRI of the head. Like a photograph that shows the features of the face, CT or MRI of the head shows the anatomy of the skull and brain. CT or MRI scans help determine whether an abnormality in the structure of the brain such as excess spinal fluid (hydrocephalus), scar tissue, or a tangle of blood vessels (vascular malformation) may be causing the epilepsy. MRI is strongly preferred over CT because it provides much more information.

A CT or MRI is usually obtained when a person has had one or more seizures to see if a structural (physical) cause is present. In the emergency room setting, a CT is often the only available test, but it can identify disorders that require urgent treatment. For most patients, an MRI should later be obtained to look for more subtle abnormalities. If a patient with partial seizures had a normal CT many years ago but the seizures persist, an MRI may provide additional information. Although one MRI is sufficient for most patients, there are exceptions. A repeat MRI scan should be considered if the cause of the seizures is known but may change (for example, a benign tumor or a vascular malformation) or if the cause is suspected but uncertain (for instance, a mild head injury). Many doctors do not order a CT or MRI for patients with well-defined epilepsy syndromes that are idiopathic (and presumably genetic), such as absence seizures, juvenile myoclonic epilepsy, or benign rolandic epilepsy, because the results are almost always normal or unrelated to epilepsy.

Several tests reveal brain function, or how it works. These methods include EEG and MEG (see above), as well as single-photon emission computed tomo-graphy (SPECT), positron emission tomography (PET), magnetic resonance spectroscopy (MRS), and functional MRI (fMRI). SPECT shows images of how much blood flows through different parts of the brain. PET shows images of how much sugar (glucose) or oxygen is metabolized, or used up, by various areas of the brain. MRS examines signals generated by elements such as carbon and phosphorus to learn about metabolic activity in the brain. fMRI measures cerebral blood flow and is used to study the neural basis of intellectual and behavioral function. All these tests are used to evaluate patients before epilepsy surgery or as research tools.

Computed Tomography

CT produces fairly good images of the brain structure (Fig. 9.8). The CT exposes the patient to low levels of radiation, although the procedure is safe, even if repeated several times. The patient's head is not in as confined a space as with MRI.

Magnetic Resonance Imaging

MRI provides detailed images of the brain's structure. (Fig. 9.9). The MRI does not use x-rays, but rather uses a powerful magnet that changes the spin on atomic particles and then measures the changes in the magnetic field as the particles resume their previous course. MRIs can identify small (as well as larger) areas of scar tissue, abnormal brain development (dysplasia), tumors, blood vessel abnormalities, and other problems.

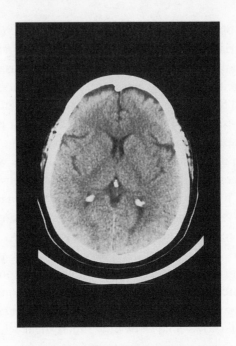

FIGURE 9.8: CT scan of a normal brain.

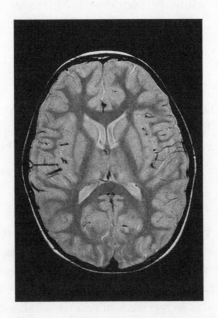

FIGURE 9.9: MRI scan of a normal brain.

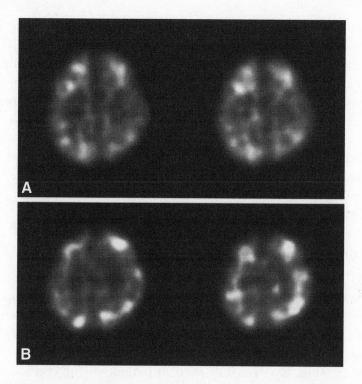

FIGURE 9.10: Two SPECT scans done on the same patient. **(A)** Interictal images (taken between seizures). **(B)** Ictal images (taken during a seizure). Bright areas on the right side of the images (in the left temporal lobe of the patient's brain) indicate increased blood flow and may mark the area from which seizure arises, called the seizure focus.

The MRI is safe and painless, but most machines confine the person's head and upper body in a small space. Persons with claustrophobia (fear of small places), and many who never knew they were claustrophobic, become frightened when they see or experience the confined space. Medications for relaxation can be given (children often require sedation), or a less confined MRI machine (open MRI) can be used, although this provides less detail. This difference can be important for patients being considered for epilepsy surgery.

Single-Photon Emission Computed Tomography

SPECT shows the blood flow in the brain. A safe, very weak radioactive compound is injected intravenously, and the particles emitted by the compound are measured. The more blood that flows through a certain area, the more particles are emitted. Available in most hospitals, for epilepsy patients, SPECT scans are mainly used as part of the surgical evaluation. SPECT scans obtained between seizures may show decreased blood flow in the seizure focus area, but the findings are often not reliable. SPECT scans obtained during a seizure are more helpful for identifying the site of seizure origin.

Computerized techniques can subtract the "between seizure" (interictal) SPECT from one taken during a seizure (ictal) to create a "subtracted" SPECT image. This image can be superimposed on the MRI to help pinpoint the seizure focus.

Positron Emission Tomography

PET, which measures the brain's metabolism of oxygen or sugar (glucose), requires the injection of a weak radioactive compound. This test is safe and helps locate the area from which partial seizures arise. PET is performed interictally, between seizures, and may show areas of decreased metabolism corresponding to the seizure focus. PET scans (Fig. 9.11) are only used in patients being considered for epilepsy surgery.

Magnetic Resonance Spectroscopy

The nuclei of certain atoms have physical qualities (resonance frequencies) that provide chemical information. MRS examines hydrogen and phosphorus atoms to determine the amounts of specific chemical compounds such as neurotransmitters and energy supplies in brain areas, providing clues to the causes and effects of epilepsy. MRS may also help to identify areas of the brain from which seizures arise, but is now considered investigational.

Lumbar Puncture

Lumbar puncture, or spinal tap, provides a sample of cerebrospinal fluid and measures pressure in the spinal canal (similar to pressure around the brain). Lumbar puncture, although not a pleasant test, has an undeservedly bad reputation as dangerous and very painful. A needle is

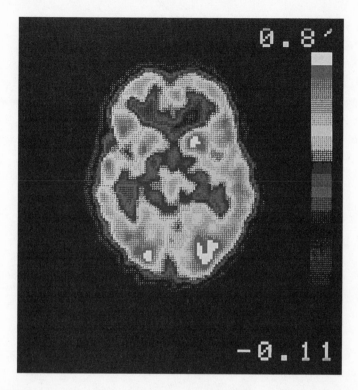

FIGURE 9.11: PET scan of the brain. PET scans use different colors (not shown) to reveal how well various areas of the brain metabolize oxygen or sugar (glucose). This metabolism is related to brain function. In this scan, for instance, differences are apparent between the functioning of the right and left temporal and parietal lobes. Normally both sides of the brain would be similar.

inserted into the sac that contains spinal fluid, several inches below the bottom of the spinal cord. For seizure patients, lumbar puncture is most often used in emergency situations to exclude bacterial meningitis or viral encephalitis.

10 | First Aid for Seizures

My little brother Bobby has seizures. Even though I babysit for other kids his age, my parents were worried to leave him with me, and I admit I was scared too. The nurse at the doctor's office helped me understand what to do if Bobby has a seizure, and my parents put a sticker on the phone with emergency phone numbers. Although I still worry that Bobby might get sick, I'll be able to do the right things to keep him safe.

K nowledge of how to respond during a seizure is essential for family members and others who are often with someone who has epilepsy. First aid is most important for tonic-clonic (convulsive) seizures. Tonic-clonic seizures—with their sudden and often unpredictable onset, falls, and convulsive movements—are frightening to witness and may appear life-threatening, but they are almost always self-limited and do not cause serious problems. A calm approach and basic first aid can minimize potential complications.

Generalized Tonic-Clonic Seizures

Generalized tonic-clonic (grand mal) seizures are convulsive seizures. The person loses consciousness, stiffens (the tonic part), falls if standing, and jerks (the clonic part). Although a convulsive seizure appears painful, the person is not conscious during the seizure. After the seizure, however, there may be discomfort caused by tongue biting, muscle soreness, headache, or bruises from falling. After the seizure, during the postictal period, the person is confused and tired. A seizure usually lasts less than 3 minutes, but that can seem like an eternity to family members or friends who watch it.

People who spend a good amount of time with someone at risk for tonic-clonic seizures should learn first-aid guidelines:

- Stay calm. Anxiety and fear are not helpful. Easy to say, hard to do.

- Help the person lie down, and place something soft under the head and neck. Keep the person (especially the head) away from sharp or hard objects such as the corner of a table.

- Time the duration of convulsive movements, if possible.

- Roll the person onto one side with the head and mouth angled toward the ground so that any excessive saliva or fluids will not accidentally be swallowed or inhaled. This position will also prevent the tongue from falling back and blocking the airway.

- Loosen all tight clothing by unfastening top shirt buttons, belts, and skirt or pant buttons. Remove any eyeglasses or tight neck chains. Do not worry about contact lenses; you could scratch the eye by trying to remove it during a seizure.

- During the convulsion, many people stop breathing (apnea) and their skin may appear bluish (cyanosis) at the peak of a seizure. As long as they start breathing again and color returns after the seizure ends, they should be fine. If regular breathing does not resume, call 911.

- Do not hold the person down; you may cause a bone dislocation or get injured yourself.

- Do not put anything in the person's mouth. The tongue cannot be swallowed during a seizure. The muscles for chewing are very strong, so a finger can be bitten, or, an object can be bitten off and the person can choke on the fragment.

🙠 After the seizure is over, do not try to restrain the person. He or she may be confused and disoriented. Restraint may provoke agitation and a violent reaction. Use a calm voice. Try to keep the person in a safe environment. Walking around is permissible, except near a street, stairs, or other potentially dangerous place.

🙠 Do not give pills, beverages, or food until the person is fully alert.

🙠 Stay with the person until he or she is fully alert and oriented. Be careful. The person may claim to be fine but still be quite confused. Ask a series of questions that require more than a yes or no answer. For example, ask "What is your address?" and "What is the date?"

🙠 Call an ambulance if any of the following occur.
1. It is the person's first tonic-clonic seizure.
2. The seizure lasts longer than 5 minutes.
3. There is more than one seizure.
4. There appears to be a significant injury (such as a head trauma or severe back pain).
5. There are problems with breathing after the seizure ends.

🙠 During and after the seizure, keep onlookers away. One or two people can provide first aid. Additional people often add confusion and embarrassment.

🙠 After the seizure is over and calm is restored, the eyewitness should tell the person who had the seizure what actually happened and the duration of the seizure and, most importantly, should provide gentle reassurance and support.

In some cases, the doctor has given other specific instructions such as rectal diazepam (see below). However, know how long to wait for seizure activity to stop after rectal diazepam is administered before calling for help.

A frequently asked question is: Does every tonic-clonic seizure require an emergency room visit? "All they do is make us wait, take blood tests and send us home with a big bill!" If the person has a history of tonic-clonic seizures, it is rarely necessary to visit the emergency room or doctor's office after a seizure unless there is an injury or the seizure was unlike previous ones. If this is the person's first tonic-clonic seizure, however, prompt medical evaluation is essential. A person with epilepsy should consider wearing a medical alert bracelet or necklace (or at a minimum, have a card in the wallet) that gives the diagnosis, medications, phone number of the doctor, and whom to call for an emergency. It can help avoid unnecessary actions and costs if a seizure occurs in a public place. MedicAlert (www.medicalert.org; 888-633-4298) is a nonprofit organization that provides bracelets, necklaces, and cards with important medical information. The organization has a 24-hour emergency response center, which provides information for emergency medical personnel. MedicAlert will also call family contacts to let them know of an emergency. Programming cell phones with ICE (In Case of Emergency) phone contact numbers is also a good idea.

A tonic-clonic seizure that lasts more than 5 minutes or a series of two or more convulsive seizures requires urgent treatment or a call for help. Drugs such as rectal diazepam (Diastat) or midazolam (not approved in the United States for this use) in the buccal space between the gum and lip can be given outside of the hospital by family members or caretakers to stop a prolonged seizure. This is especially important for patients with a history of prolonged or recurrent convulsions and for those who live far from a hospital or who are traveling to remote areas (e.g., camping). The doses of these drugs should be carefully reviewed with the physician, including if and when a second dose may be given if seizure activity persists.

The patient is best transported to a medical facility by ambulance, as he or she may need oxygen or medication and a convulsion in a passenger car can be dangerous for everyone. How long does a seizure have to last to warrant a call for help? There is no absolute answer; discuss it with the doctor. In general, if the convulsion lasts more than 5 minutes, or if the need for assistance is uncertain, call for help.

Seizures may cause bruises, cuts, sprains, or a bitten tongue, but they rarely cause broken or dislocated bones (most often the shoulder) or other more serious problems. After the seizure, the person may complain of headache, mouth discomfort from tongue- or cheek-biting, or back pain related to the muscular contractions or a fall. Acetaminophen (Tylenol) or ibuprofen (Advil, Motrin) is helpful for minor pains. If back pain is severe, a doctor should be consulted to assess for a fracture, which is usually treated conservatively with rest. Fever may follow a seizure, usually because of the muscle activity and the effects of the seizure.

If the fever is unusually high (over 102°F), lasts more than 3 hours, or develops more than 2 hours after a seizure, it is wise to consult with a doctor. Sometimes secretions or food goes down the respiratory tract during the seizure and cause pneumonia.

Atonic and Tonic Seizures

Atonic seizures (sudden loss of muscle strength) and tonic seizures (suddenly stiffening) often cause sudden falls with a high potential for injury. Because the fall may occur at or within a few seconds of seizure onset, it may be impossible to prevent. Occasionally, the occurrence or increased frequency of other seizure types (such as absence or myoclonic seizures) is a warning that an atonic or tonic seizure is about to happen and the person can sit or lie down. Patients who have atonic or tonic seizures without warning need protective headgear that may need to include a facemask to prevent injury. Both Danmar helmets, made especially for this, and Cooper hockey helmets provide good protection.

Complex Partial Seizures

Complex partial seizures are rarely associated with injury unless the person is driving or operating dangerous equipment. Single and brief complex partial seizures do not damage the brain. Prolonged or repetitive complex partial seizures may cause slight but persistent memory loss.

During a complex partial seizure, speak quietly and in a reassuring manner, because some persons can react to emotional or physical stimulation. Do not yell at the person or restrain him or her unless absolutely necessary, which is rare. Keep the person safe from harm. For example, burns can occur when someone unknowingly touches or falls on a hot object. During and after some complex partial seizures, the person may walk or rarely run without a good sense of his or her environment. When this occurs near dangerous equipment, a busy city street, train tracks, or high places, there is a potential for serious injury.

Other behaviors during complex partial seizures may cause concern, but are not dangerous. These include screaming, kicking, ripping up papers, disrobing, sexual-like movements, and, rarely, masturbation.

If someone has unusual automatisms, he or she should be led in a quiet and reassuring manner out of public places, such as an office or store. Strategies should be devised to minimize the embarrassing effects of unusual seizures.

The greatest danger occurs when the person is driving a car or operating dangerous equipment. Those with seizures that impair consciousness or control of movement should avoid these activities.

If the seizure is prolonged (more than 5 minutes) or if there are three or more complex partial seizures, then medical help should be sought. Rectal diazepam (Diastat), buccal midazolam, or sublingual lorazepam (Ativan) can be administered at home by family members to stop the seizures. First aid for someone having a complex partial seizure is simple:

- Keep the person away from dangerous situations.

- Use restraint only if it is necessary for his or her safety.

- Seek medical help for prolonged (>5 minutes) or recurrent seizures.

Simple Partial Seizures

Simple partial seizures rarely require first aid. Since consciousness is preserved, the person is almost always aware of the seizure and the surroundings. When simple partial seizures progress to complex partial or secondarily generalized tonic-clonic seizures, the person should be quietly and cautiously moved to a safe environment and should stop driving or working with dangerous equipment.

Absence Seizures

Absence seizures usually require no first aid. They are brief and are almost never associated with falling or injury. If absence seizures occur in a cluster, it may be wise to remove a child from sports, swimming, or other potentially dangerous activities *during the cluster period*. Very rarely, absence seizures can occur as a continuous state (absence status epilepticus). If this happens, medications can be given by mouth, under the tongue (sublingual), between the lip and gum (buccal) or rectum to stop the seizure, or medical attention should be sought.

11 | Principles of Drug Therapy for Epilepsy

Antiepileptic drugs (AEDs) are the principal therapy for epilepsy. Choosing an effective drug depends on correctly diagnosing the type of epilepsy (generalized versus partial) and, ideally, the epilepsy syndrome. Next, a decision whether or not to treat needs to be made. For most patients, the benefits of AEDs and seizure control outweigh the risks. Finally, there are the big questions—what drug to choose and what to do next if it doesn't work or isn't tolerated?

There is rarely one best drug. In most cases, several AEDs are similar in effectiveness but have different side effects. A patient and his or her doctor should discuss the pros and cons of each drug. For example, relevant medication issues include frequency of dosing (most patients prefer once or twice a day), side effects (tiredness, weight gain or loss), safety risks, cost, and potential risks during pregnancy. The next chapter reviews individual AEDs.

Although AEDs control seizures in most people, they do not cure epilepsy. People often remark, "These drugs don't really treat the epilepsy, they just control seizures. They are like Band-Aids." There is truth in that statement. If scar tissue or an abnormal group of blood vessels in the brain causes seizures, AEDs will surely not repair these structural problems. These medications suppress seizures but do not "fix" the underlying cause. However, the longer someone is seizure-free while taking AEDs, the better the chances he or she will remain seizure-free when the medications are stopped.

Goals of Drug Therapy

The goals of AED therapy are simple: no seizures, no side effects. Many people can reach these goals easily, but for others, the balance between seizure control and side effects is delicate and compromises are unavoidable. Communication between the doctor and the patient is critical to reach optimal treatment. The patient and the doctor should openly discuss what to expect, what is tolerable, what the patient is experiencing, and the impact of side effects and seizures on quality of life.

Do not accept troublesome side effects without finding out if they are avoidable. Some patients fear that if they complain about a medication, the doctor will reduce it and a seizure will occur or because they believe that side effects are a necessary evil (which they sometimes are). Many people who take medications for long periods are unable to separate a side effect from "who they are." Some doctors may incorrectly label complaints as psychological or due to other factors, especially if the patient is on low doses of medication or the doctor is not familiar with the side effect. Some people are extremely sensitive to medications and experience problems on low dosages. Others incorrectly blame every minor problem on a new drug. The best way to sort out these issues is by carefully observing the potential side effects—how soon did they begin after initiation or increase in a medication? Do they often occur at a similar time after a drug is taken? How long do they last? What makes them better?

Changes in medications should be done systematically and be limited to one drug at a time whenever possible. This strategy helps establish a relationship between a change and an effect such as improved seizure control or worsening side effect.

Time Required for Antiepileptic Drugs to Work

Absorption

Oral medication passes through the stomach and is absorbed in the small intestine. It may then go to the liver, where many drugs are metabolized or broken down, and then enters into the bloodstream. Eventually, AEDs reach the brain. Some drugs are mainly eliminated by the kidneys in an unchanged (not metabolized) form.

Peak Effect

An oral dose of medication will reach a peak, or maximum, blood level after 30 minutes to 6 hours. The time between taking the medication and reaching the peak level depends on the specific drug, its form (liquid, tablet, capsule, slow-release form), and, in some cases, the food consumed before taking it. The properties of selected AEDs when used as sole therapy are summarized in Table 12.1.

I felt like I might have a seizure, so I took an extra pill

This commonsense approach often fails to prevent a seizure. In most cases, when a person experiences an aura, progression to a larger seizure occurs in seconds or a few minutes. Since most medicines take more than 10–15 minutes to begin reaching the brain, oral medications will rarely stop an imminent seizure. However, if the person feels vulnerable to a seizure over the coming hours, this approach could reduce the risk of a seizure—for example, a person who is sleep deprived and feels his or her "brain is not working right" and recalls this feeling 30–60 minutes before prior seizures. In many cases, a more rapidly acting medicine such as lorazepam may be used to try and prevent an approaching seizure.

Half–Life

The goal with AEDs is to maintain a relatively constant level in the blood. A drug's *half-life* is time required for the drug's peak concentration in the blood to drop by 50% (Fig. 11.1).

Some drugs, such as carbamazepine, gabapentin, levetiracetam, pregabalin, and tiagabine, have a relatively short half-life (<10 hours); some, such as lamotrigine, topiramate, and phenytoin, have an intermediate half-life (~24 hours); and some, such as phenobarbital and zonisamide, have a long half-life (>40 hours) (see Chapter 12). Different preparations of the same drugs often have different times to peak level and half-life. For example, carbamazepine is available as a generic tablet, brand-name tablet (Tegretol), chewable brand-name tablet (Tegretol), brand-name sustained-release tablet (Tegretol XR) or capsule (Carbatrol), and elixir (liquid). Each form has a different half-life. Because of these differences in absorption and half-life, switching to a rapidly absorbed or shorter half-life form can cause a higher peak level (more side effects) and seizures (lower end-of dose [trough] blood levels, risk of seizure). When drugs are used in combination, the half-life of each drug may change.

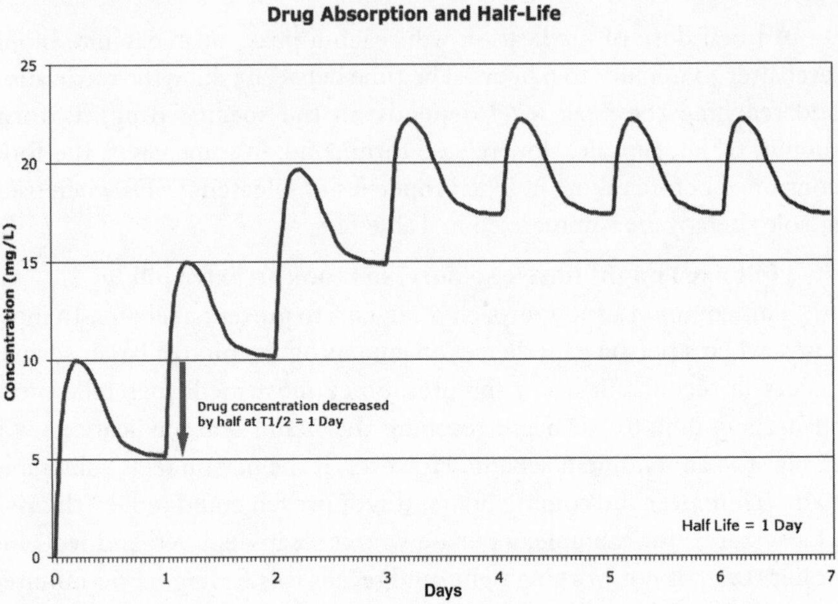

Drug Absorption and Half-Life

FIGURE 11.1: Drug absorption and half-life.

In general, half-lives are shortest in children, intermediate in adults, and longest in the elderly. Also, elixirs are usually more rapidly absorbed and therefore have shorter half-lives. Products with delayed absorption or release have longer half-lives. Drugs in forms that have gradual release and gradual absorption are ideal, as they produce steadier blood drug levels. Then doses can be taken less often without wide swings in the blood levels.

Drugs with longer half-lives have more stable blood levels and need to be taken less frequently. Drugs with short half-lives ideally should be taken several times a day to prevent adverse effects during periods of high blood levels and seizures during periods of low levels. Occasionally, drugs with short half-lives can be taken less frequently, because the effect on the brain is long-lasting.

Steady State

Steady state (equilibrium) is when blood drug levels are fairly constant on a constant dosage. Thus, steady state is when the amount of drug taken and the amount being metabolized and excreted are equal. It takes approximately fives times longer than the half-life of the drug to arrive at equilibrium (Fig. 11.1).

Even at equilibrium, the levels will fluctuate over the course of the day and from day to day. Depending on the rate of absorption and the factors that influence the absorption rate (for example, taking some drugs after meals slows absorption), there will be peaks in the blood level within hours after the drug is taken and troughs (low points) shortly before or immediately after a dose is taken, especially if there is a long interval between doses. Fluctuations between the peak level and the trough level depend mainly on the half-life of the drug (short half-life means greater fluctuation) and the number of times the medication is taken each day (if a drug has a short half-life, taking it frequently will reduce the fluctuations). Dose-related side effects are more likely to occur at peak levels, and a seizure is more likely to occur with trough levels. Blood levels can also be influenced by other medications, viral infections, menstrual cycle, and other factors.

I vomited after I took my pill, should I take another?

Absorption woes: Vomiting and Diarrhea—Beware! A majority of epilepsy patients who sleep well, take their medication regularly, and consume little or no alcohol will be seizure-free. However, vomiting and diarrhea can reduce the absorption of medication, lowering blood levels and possibly causing seizures, especially in the setting of an illness.

The interval between oral intake and absorption varies. When gastrointestinal (GI) function is abnormal, as occurs with a GI virus or food poisoning, two common causes of vomiting and diarrhea, absorption can be delayed and reduced. Therefore, lthough most tablets are absorbed within a few hours, in the setting of a GI illness, it can take much longer. If pill fragments are seen in the vomitus, the medicine was probably not absorbed. If the illness is prolonged, repeating the dose may not fix the problem since absorption is still impaired. In such cases, a medicine such as lorazepam under the tongue may be an effective short-term solution until the GI function returns to normal.

Diarrhea causes more rapid passage of medicines through the GI system. This can impair absorption and lower blood levels. If diarrhea is watery and occurs for more than 4–6 hours, you should notify your physician and consider a temporary increase in medication dosage to help prevent a seizure.

How consistent do I have to be with my meds? If I give it to my daughter an hour late, could it cause a seizure?

For the vast majority of patients, taking a medication up to 2 hours before or after the regular time will not cause seizures or side effects. Indeed, a single missed dose of medication is very unlikely to cause a seizure—but it does significantly increase the risk! Try to be consistent about the timing of medication and food—this helps avoid missed doses that can lead to seizures, as well side effects from doses that are too close together.

Adverse Effects of AEDs

Doctors and patients with epilepsy see medical care from different perspectives. The doctor would like to see the patient regularly, have the patient take medication regularly, and have the patient's seizures well controlled. The patient would like never to see a doctor, never to take a pill, and have the seizures go away. Patients often consider taking pills even worse than seeing a doctor.

AED side effects can be minor or severe, short-lasting and reversible, or long-lasting and, very rarely, irreversible (see Table 12.2). Most are mild and transient. Before starting a medication, the patient should know what to expect. Some fatigue, abdominal discomfort, or dizziness is common during the first weeks taking an AED, but if the medication is started at a low dosage and increased slowly, and if the patient is aware of what to expect, these effects are usually tolerable. They usually stop after several weeks or months, as tolerance develops.

Side effects are broadly divided into two types: those that are unpredictable and are not related to dosage or blood level (*idiosyncratic*) and those that are related to the dose and blood level (*dose-related*).

Idiosyncratic Effects

Idiosyncratic side effects include rash, fever, inflammation of the liver or pancreas, and a serious reduction in the number of white blood cells (immune system), platelets (control bleeding), and red blood cells (carry oxygen). Dangerous but very rare idiosyncratic reactions such as aplastic anemia (severe damage to bone marrow causing a failure in the production of blood cells) and liver failure are allergic reactions, and usually occur within the first year of starting a drug. Other idiosyncratic side effects include hair loss, swollen lymph glands, or ulcers or white spots in the mouth.

If a rash or fever develops after a new medication is prescribed, call the doctor immediately. The doctor will have to decide if the rash is a drug-related (allergic) rash or an unrelated rash. Drug rashes usually begin 5–18 days after a medication is started. Allergic reactions may start with fever and/or swollen glands and the rash emerges several days later. Many rashes are mild and may be unrelated to the drug. For example, rash can result from viruses, bacteria, allergic reactions, laundry detergent, insect bites, and other causes. In persons taking more than one drug, the one that was most recently started has probably caused the rash. The drug-related rash usually resolves shortly after the medication is discontinued. Some side effects of medication can be serious, but life-threatening problems are extremely rare. Fewer than 1 person in 75,000 who take AEDs will die as a result; the chance of dying in a motor vehicle accident is much greater. The more serious risks include rashes that cause peeling of the skin or involve mucous membranes (for example, the mouth), infection from a low white blood cell count, serious bleeding from a low platelet count, liver damage, or pancreas damage. Less serious, but potentially problematic risks include kidney stones, significant weight gain, gum overgrowth, drop in blood sodium, and neuropathy. In almost every case, when a doctor recommends treatment, the benefits of AEDs outweigh the risks. *Persons who have excessive bleeding, abdominal pain and tenderness, fever, unusual infections, or other unusual symptoms while taking a drug should tell their doctor immediately.*

Dose-Related Effects

Toxicity

Dose-related side effects are more common than idiosyncratic effects. When the dosage of a drug is increased, the blood level may become too high for the person to tolerate, and troublesome effects, called *toxicity*, will occur. It is difficult to predict the exact dosage or blood level of a drug that will cause toxicity in a given person.

Common dose-related side effects are dizziness, tiredness, stomach discomfort, headache, tremor, unsteadiness, irritability, mild depression, and blurred or double vision. At higher or toxic dosage, more severe forms of all these problems can occur, as well as cognitive impairment, vomiting, diarrhea, and psychosis. These are side effects related to drug dose which may be short term and resolved with lower doses.

Metabolites may contribute to toxicity. Most metabolites are *inactive*, but some drugs such as carbamazepine and valproate produce *active metabolites*—substances derived from the liver's "digestion"—that can have antiepileptic and side effects of their own. Measuring only blood levels of carbamazepine or valproate may be misleading, as the metabolite may be contributing to the problem. Other drugs can also alter the level of active metabolites.

Side effects from medication (other than "idiosyncratic" ones), including toxicity, are almost never dangerous or permanent. By spreading the total dose more evenly (or frequently) throughout the day, having the patient take medications with meals or at bedtime, or lowering the dose, the doctor can usually alleviate abdominal discomfort, blurred vision, headache, or fatigue.

I wasn't sure so I didn't mention it

We all hope that if we ignore something, it will go away. Common side effects, such as dizziness or tiredness, that occur shortly after a medication is started, are often transient and mild. However, patients should report any unusual symptoms to their doctor, especially during the first 8 weeks after starting a new AED. For example, a new fever or rash could be a serious side effect and may require the doctor to stop the new AED. Alternatively, some patients come in with a multipage list of problems that encompass many minor issues that could prevent the doctor from recognizing important problems.

If I stay on this medication for 5 or 10 years, won't it eventually destroy my liver or kidneys?

No! Unlike chronic excessive alcohol intake that can progressively damage liver function, AEDs do not have a similar effect. Long-lasting adverse effects, such as nerve damage from phenytoin, are uncommon. The major exception is bone loss (see below).

I have heard that seizure medicines thin your bones

Bone loss from certain AEDs is more common than generally appreciated by doctors and patients. Patients taking drugs that increase the activity of certain liver enzymes—carbamazepine, phenobarbital,

Table 11.1. Antiepileptic Drugs That May Aggravate Seizures

Drug	Seizure type affected
Carbamazepine	Absence, myoclonic, BRE, JME, LGS
Ethosuximide	Myoclonic, tonic-clonic
Gabapentin	Absence, myoclonic, LGS
Lamotrigine	Myoclonic, atonic, JME, LGS, BRE
Oxcarbazepine	Absence, myoclonic, JME, LGS
Phenytoin	Absence, myoclonic, JME, LGS
Tiagabine	Absence
Vigabatrin[a]	Absence, myoclonic, LGS

BRE, benign rolandic epilepsy; JME, juvenile myoclonic epilepsy; LGS, Lennox-Gastaut syndrome.
[a] Not FDA-approved.

phenytoin, primidone, topiramate, or valproate—should consider taking calcium and vitamin D supplements and obtaining bone density measurements.

Someone told me their seizures were made worse by their seizure medication!

AEDs can occasionally worsen seizures (Table 11.1). The best protection is to keep a log of medication dosage and seizures. If an increase in dosage is associated with an increase in seizures, the doctor should be notified. However, seizure frequency varies with many factors. Be careful not to confuse correlation with causation. For example, low doses of a new medicine may be associated with an increased seizure frequency that is either coincidental or a result of lowering another medication. The medicine may be very effective for the patient, but the dosage is actually too low.

Cognitive Effects

AEDs often reduce the excitability of brain cells. They can also dampen normal activity and impair cognitive function—aspects such as attention and concentration, memory, mood, drive (e.g., "will to do things"), and mental and motor speed on tests (see Chapter 11).

Cognitive impairments are more likely when two or more drugs are used (*polytherapy*) and when blood levels exceed the therapeutic range. Reducing the number of drugs or dosage can help improve cognition. However, some patients are sensitive and may experience cognitive problems on a single drug whose blood level is "therapeutic". Phenobarbital, primidone, and topiramate are associated with increased rates of cognitive problems.

I have been on phenobarbital for years and have no side effects

These were the words of a woman who was evaluated for surgery. Prior to her temporal lobectomy, she was changed from phenobarbital to levetiracetam. Her employer called to speak to me (after she gave permission)—"she gained 50 IQ points!" Although he overstated her improvement, she was much brighter with improved memory, mental processing speed, and mood. If a drug has been used for years, it is often impossible to assess side effects.

A person's subjective perception of cognitive side effects lessens over time more than their perception of physical side effects. Sadly, it seems that we are more likely to accommodate to slowed mental function than to a stomach ache or blurred vision. The subjective perception of cognitive performance is often related to mood as well as performance. Thus, when a patient complains about cognitive side effects, it often correlates more with depression or sadness (dysphoria) than cognitive impairment. The patient, family, and doctor must therefore be vigilant on two fronts: (1) to identify cognitive impairment resulting from AEDs (especially certain AEDs and high doses or polytherapy), as well as (2) to identify depression. Seeking objective measures of cognitive performance such as school grades, input from relatives, neuropsychological testing, and assessment of mood can help clarify the underlying cause(s).

Behavioral Effects

AEDs can cause problems with anxiety, irritability, or depression; rarely, mania (abnormally elevated mood, energy, and activity), paranoia, or psychosis can occur. Behavioral problems are usually mild and transient, but can occasionally be severe and chronic. They can be reversed by lowering the dose or discontinuing the AED. It is difficult to predict who will develop behavioral side effects, although people with prior psychiatric disorders and developmental delays may be moresusceptible. Behavioral problems are more common when a drug dose is rapidly increased, if high doses are used, or multiple AEDs (polytherapy). Levetiracetam, phenobarbital, mysoline, topiramate, vigabatrin, and zonisamide are associated with increased rates of behavioral problems. Gabapentin has been associated with behavioral problems in children.

Can I become addicted to my medication?

No! In the vast majority of cases, AEDs have no addictive potential. Some patients fear that once they start taking a medication, they may become "hooked." There is no medical basis for this fear. The only AEDs with addictive potential are benzodiazepines (clonazepam, clorazepate, and lorazepam, clobazam) and barbiturates (phenobarbital, primidone). Addiction to benzodiazepines or barbiturates is rare in adolescents and adults and does not occur in children with epilepsy.

Benzodiazepines and barbiturates can be successfully discontinued, but it must be done gradually to avoid seizures and other withdrawal symptoms such as rapid heart rate, sweating, and anxiety. Withdrawal symptoms occur even when the drug is tapered gradually, especially if the medication has been used for a long time.

Tolerance

Tolerance is the body's response to the repeated administration of a specific drug (or class of drugs) that decreases the medication's effect. Thus, the drug becomes less potent over time and larger doses must be used to obtain the same effect, whether the effect is good (seizure control) or bad (sleepiness, for instance). There are two main forms of tolerance. *Metabolic tolerance* is more effective elimination of the drug (for example, more rapid liver metabolism). Pharmacodynamic tolerance is an adaptive change in the tissue or organ affected by the drug. For example, long-term use of benzodiazepines reduces the sensitivity of the gamma-amino butyric acid (GABA) receptors, so a given dose of the drug is less effective. Regularly using one drug of this type (for example, clonazepam taken by mouth) will produce tolerance to another type (such as rectal diazepam).

A very small amount of tolerance can occur for most AEDs, but it usually does not affect seizure control. Occasionally, patients do well with a new drug for several weeks or months, but the drug becomes less effective over time and seizures recur or become more frequent (the "honeymoon effect").

Benzodiazepines are the AEDs most often associated with clinically significant tolerance. These drugs are among the most powerful in the emergency control of prolonged seizures, but they are much less effective in long-term treatment.

Missed Doses

People on long-term medication sometimes forget a dose. For example, someone may oversleep and, in the rush to get to work, forget the morning medication, or she may simply fall asleep before taking the bedtime dose. Given the differences in epilepsy type and seizure control between patients as well as the variations in drug half-lives and other factors, ask your doctor what to do if you miss one or more doses of medication. As a general rule, if a single dose is missed, I recommend that it be taken as soon as possible. Avoid "doubling up" on the next dose, as this may lead to side effects; instead, take the missed dose as soon as possible and then take the next scheduled dose after an interval of at least 2 hours, often with some food to delay the second dose's absorption.

If two doses are missed within the same 24-hour period, it is usually recommended that one dose be taken as soon as it is remembered and the second missed dose 2–4 hours later. If more than two doses of medication are missed in one 24-hour period, or if medication is missed entirely for more than 24 hours, the doctor's office should be called.

No, that can't be the cause of the seizure, I've missed a lot of doses

A 45-year-old man with rare nocturnal seizures who was on lamotrigine 300 mg once daily called after a tonic-clonic seizure during breakfast. He was devastated because his children saw the seizure and afraid to drive. "How could this happen?" he asked. My first question was if he missed his medication in the past few days. He said yes, but was convinced this could not be the cause, since he had often missed doses. I explained that missing a dose was like gambling. No matter how good the odds are, if you do it enough, you will probably lose!

Table 11.2. Primary and Secondary AEDs for Different Seizure Types and Epilepsy Syndromes

Seizure type	Primary drug	Secondary drug
Idiopathic (Primary) Generalized		
Absence	Ethosuximide Lamotrigine Valproate	Zonisamide Topiramate
Myoclonic	Valproate Levetiracetam	Clonazepam Lamotrigine Topiramate Zonisamide
Tonic-clonic	Valproate Lamotrigine Topiramate Levetiracetam	Carbamazepine Oxcarbazepine Phenytoin Zonisamide
Juvenile myoclonic epilepsy syndrome	Valproate Lamotrigine Levetiracetam	Acetazolamide Clonazepam Primidone Topiramate
Infantile spasms (West syndrome)	Adrenocorticotropic hormone (ACTH) Vigabatrin	Topiramate Valproate
Lennox-Gastaut syndrome	Valproate Lamotrigine Topirmate	Carbamazepine Oxcarbazepine Felbamate Zonisamide
Partial		
Simple partial, complex partial, and secondary generalized tonic-clonic seizures	Carbamazepine Lamotrigine Levetiracetam Oxcarbazepine Zonisamide	Gabapentin Phenytoin Pregabalin Topiramate Valproate
Benign epilepsy of childhood with centro-temporal spikes (BECTS)	Carbamazepine Lamotrigine Oxcarbazepine	Levetiracetam Gabapentin Pregabalin Topiramate Valproate Zonisamide

Drug Absorption and Food

All AEDs can be taken around meal time. A full stomach delays, but does not reduce absorption. Side effects due to peak levels, such as blurred vision or dizziness, may be reduced by taking the medicine during or after meals to slow absorption. Peak side effects are most common 30 minutes to several hours after a dose.

Primary AEDs

The effectiveness of each AED varies by seizure type. For each type of seizure, one or more drugs may be considered the "best" based on effectiveness and mild side effect profile. One of these "best" drugs is usually recommended as a first-line treatment for the patient's main type of seizure (Table 11.2). Because some medications work well for certain seizure types but are ineffective or may worsen other types, correct diagnosis is essential. In prescribing AEDs, doctors usually start with just one drug, beginning with a low dose and increasing it slowly unless the patient's condition requires a more rapid build-up. The correct dosage is based on how well the patient is doing (Are seizures controlled? Are there adverse effects?), not on the amount of drug in the patient's blood.

Many patients have several types of seizure. For example, a patient with juvenile myoclonic epilepsy may have myoclonic and tonic-clonic seizures. Lamotrigine may be well tolerated and effective in controlling tonic-clonic seizures but have little effect on, or even increase the frequency of, the myoclonic seizures. In such cases, the benefits of lamotrigine may outweigh the costs, or it may be preferable to find a medication that controls all seizure types.

In general, AEDs are most effective for severe seizures (tonic-clonic seizures), intermediate in effectiveness for moderate intensity seizures (complex partial seizures), and least effective in fully controlling mild seizures (simple partial seizures). For patients with partial epilepsy who suffer from different strength seizures, there is no evidence that one drug targets complex partial while another targets simple partial or secondarily generalized tonic-clonic seizures. Rather, if a drug works against partial epilepsy, it works against all seizure types. There may be individual exceptions to this rule.

Patients find it easiest to take one small pill once a day. The size and number of the pills may not reflect the drug's effectiveness or adverse effects. If 100 mg of drug A has the same beneficial effect as 10 mg (a much smaller pill) of drug B, then drug B is more potent. For example, a patient taking 150 mg of phenobarbital once at bedtime may experience both better seizure control and fewer side effects if gradually changed to 750 mg levetiracetam two times daily, although the amount of drug taken, the size of the pills, and the frequency of dose are all increased. The first goal should be seizure control with minimal or no side effects. The number and size of the pills are important, but secondary issues.

In most patients, a single primary AED provides the best balance between seizure control and side effects. Unfortunately, some patients are treated with three or more AEDs, at moderate doses, and suffer both seizures and side effects. This is not a good strategy. If seizures persist while a patient is taking a single medication that causes no side effects, it is usually best to increase the dose until the seizures are controlled or side effects develop. Rapid dose increases can cause side effects and unnecessarily lead to disabling fatigue, impaired concentration, or other problems that are considered "necessary" side effects of the drug. With many drugs, the key to tolerability is a gradual increase in the dosage. Some patients may require two or even three medications to gain full control of seizures. In these cases, the benefits should outweigh the risks.

AEDs vary considerably in how they work, how long they remain in the blood (half-life), and how they should be taken (specific drugs are reviewed in Chapter 12). Patients should not experiment with varying the schedule of their medications without first discussing the proposed changes with the doctor or nurse. Because some medications, such as gabapentin, have short half-lives, they almost always have to be taken more than once a day to control seizures and minimize side effects.

The schedule for taking medication should be flexible and adapted to the patient's lifestyle. In most cases, it is easy for the doctor and patient to work out a schedule that is convenient, minimizes adverse effects, and controls seizures.

Secondary AEDs

A rash, disabling fatigue, or other problems may force the doctor to stop the first AED. In these cases, another primary drug is usually tried alone. If the first primary drug is tolerated and blood levels are in the high therapeutic range but it fails to control the seizures, some experts will try another primary or *secondary* drug alone while others will recommend adding another drug to the regimen (see Table 11.2). When one medication is added to another medication, it is referred to as *adjunctive therapy*. Use of one medicine is *monotherapy*, while two or more drugs is called *polytherapy*. Although some drugs are called *secondary* because they tend to have fewer good effects and more bad effects than the primary drugs, secondary drugs can be very safe and effective. Many patients are successfully treated using only secondary drugs.

What If the Drug Fails?

The first attempt at AED therapy may be ineffective for several reasons:

- It is the wrong drug for the patient's seizure type or epilepsy syndrome.
- The patient didn't take the medication as prescribed.
- The prescribed doses didn't control the seizures.
- The patient had an allergic reaction (such as rash or hives) to the medication.
- The patient experienced side medication effects such as tiredness or nausea.

Can the diagnosis of seizure type or epilepsy syndrome be wrong? Yes! It happens to all doctors—primary care doctors, general neurologists, and epilepsy experts. Misinterpretation of the clinical history or EEG is usually responsible. Clinical history can be contaminated by leading questions (that may falsely evoke a positive response) or false conclusions. Also, dogma misleads doctors.

A common reason for a drug to fail is missed doses, which cause a breakthrough seizure in someone who was previously controlled. How does one find the correct dosage? This is the "lowest effective dose"—the least amount of medication that protects the patient against seizures, even during periods of stress or sleep deprivation (which are impossible to fully avoid) or the occasional missed dose. Less than this can result in breakthrough seizures, while more can result in side effects. The "right" dose cannot be determined ahead of time, but depends on individual factors such as absorption and metabolism of medication, severity of epilepsy, and lifestyle.

A drug may fail if the medication doses are not timed correctly, and low levels occur when seizures are most likely. During the circadian day-wake cycle, seizures may occur randomly or at similar times. For those with random seizures, therapeutic levels should be maintained continuously. For people prone to seizures at specific times, doses can be timed to maximize seizure control and minimize side effects. If seizures only occur shortly before or after awakening, the largest, or only, dose should be given at bedtime. For a child with benign rolandic epilepsy who has only had seizures within an hour after falling asleep, a single daily dose several hours before bedtime may be effective and minimize daytime side effects. Finally, a drug may simply fail because it is ineffective.

Allergic reactions usually require that the drug be discontinued. Dose-related side effects can often be managed by decreasing the dose temporarily until the patient becomes more "used to the drug" (until tolerance develops). In other cases, giving small doses more often, giving the medication after meals, or giving a larger dose at bedtime may reduce side effects.

If intolerable side effects occur even with low doses, the drug should be discontinued and another drug should be tried. If relatively high doses and "therapeutic" blood levels of a drug fail to control seizures, try another single drug or two drugs. The decision should be based on the potential benefits and side effects of one versus two drugs. If a second drug is added, track the change in seizure frequency and severity as well as side effects with different dosages. Do the benefits of the second drug outweigh additional side effects and financial cost? For example, a 20% reduction in seizure frequency may not be worth the cost of severe tiredness and dizziness.

If two different drugs given singly and a combination of two drugs fail to control seizures, all at dosages that yield blood levels in the therapeutic range, the chances that another drug or combination of drugs will fully control the seizures are less than 15%. Before trying other medications, it is often worth consulting with an epilepsy specialist to ensure that the diagnosis and medication selection are correct. If seizures are not easily controllable with medication, it may be worth exploring the possibility of the ketogenic or modified Atkins diet, epilepsy surgery, or vagus nerve stimulation.

Blood Testing

Blood tests should be done before any AED is started so that the results can be compared with later blood tests. These tests include measurements of electrolyte levels (such as sodium and potassium), liver and kidney function tests, and blood cell counts.

Once a medication is started, blood tests may be obtained to determine if there are abnormalities in these measurements and/or to determine the level of medication in the blood.

How often should blood tests be obtained?

There are two issues—one is on obtaining metabolic tests (liver enzymes, sodium level, etc.) and blood cell counts to screen for very, very rare (less than 1 per 20,000) but potentially life-threatening problems. Routine blood screens for such disorders are not warranted. Baseline tests should be obtained before a drug is started and may need to be rechecked if new problems arise (such as serious infection or bleeding) or if seizures increase for no apparent reason. More often, metabolic or blood cell abnormalities will be found (e.g., low sodium in patients taking oxcarbazepine) that are clinically insignificant or require a change in therapy.

The second issue concerns monitoring the drug's blood level. There are two views and no right answer. One says "treat the patient, not the laboratory studies." The other says "more information is better." Many American neurologists, especially those who treat adults, obtain screening blood and follow-up tests and drug levels more often than European neurologists. They decrease the dose if patients have bothersome side effects, regardless of the blood level. For European doctors, blood levels should be monitored only if unexplained seizures occur or if they are not sure that the patient takes the drug as prescribed.

A middle road seems reasonable, but most importantly, decisions about blood testing should be individually tailored. I recommend blood tests before and 2–10 weeks after a medication is started. After that, it depends on how the patient is doing. For those who have no seizures and no side effects, tests may be obtained once a year or not at all. For those with ongoing seizures but no side effects, the dosage of medication can be increased without checking the levels. However, it is often worth checking to that there is not a problem with the patient taking their medication, absorption, metabolism, or drug interactions that could affect the medication levels.

Drug levels should be checked at consistent times of day and consistent times after the last dose of medication was taken. This allows the doctor to compare levels at different dosages. Routine blood levels are best measured when the amount of the drug is at its lowest point, the trough level. This generally corresponds to the time just before the medication is taken. Trough levels fluctuate up to 15–20% in many patients who take the drug on a consistent schedule. These variations reflect changes in the drug's absorption and metabolism, other medications taken, and handling of the blood specimen at the laboratory.

The therapeutic range of blood levels for AEDs is overrated and overused. This statistical concept, derived from patients, often fails for the individual patient. The therapeutic range approximates where most patients have good seizure control and few side effects. The lower and upper limits of this range can vary between different laboratories and doctors. Seizure control without side effects, not the blood drug level, determines the right dose. For example, if a patient's seizures are well controlled but the level of drug in the blood is below the "therapeutic range," the dose is probably fine. For a patient whose seizures only came under control with a high dosage of medication that produced blood levels slightly above the therapeutic level (in the "toxic range") with very minor side effects, the drug dosage should probably not be decreased.

Unless seizures or side effects are a problem, blood levels do not need to be monitored regularly (and many would say at all!). In some cases, however, it may be critical to attain a therapeutic blood drug level. It may be necessary to check blood levels before and after adding or removing another medication (including medications taken for conditions other than epilepsy), due to the possibility of drug interactions (see below). As another example, a pregnant woman on lamotrigine should have blood levels checked monthly since on steady doses, blood levels often decline by more than 50% (see Chapter 26).

Drug Interactions

A doctor caring for a person with epilepsy should know about all of the drugs the person is taking. Drug interactions are common and can be dangerous. AEDs may interact with each other and with other drugs. Drug interactions can decrease blood levels of the antiepileptic or other drug, leading to seizures or other problems. Blood levels can also increase, leading to toxicity.

No list of drug interactions is all-inclusive, as doctors and pharmacists continue to learn of interactions between existing drugs and new ones. Therefore, the doctor or other health care provider who prescribes medication for a person with epilepsy should be aware that he or she is taking an AED. Patients should also tell the pharmacist or doctor about their use of over-the-counter medications because some of them can affect AED levels, cause seizures in someone who has never had a seizure, or increase seizure frequency in a person with epilepsy. The tables in Appendix C list drug interactions involving AEDs. A Google search can also be helpful, but sources vary widely on the Internet so use reliable sources (e.g., www.epilepsy.com).

AEDs and Birth Control Pills

Most women with epilepsy can take birth control pills without affecting their seizure control. Usually there is no change when the pills are started, though some women have slightly improved or worsened seizure control. Some AEDs (carbamazepine, oxcarbazepine, phenytoin, phenobarbital, primidone, and topiramate) increase the breakdown, or metabolism, of estrogen and progesterone by the liver, and reduce the effectiveness of birth control pills. If a sexually active woman is taking birth control pills and one of these drugs, she should be aware that her chances of getting pregnant are increased.

Breakthrough bleeding between menstrual periods is a clue that the effectiveness of birth control pills is reduced. However, the absence of breakthrough bleeding does not indicate that the woman has adequate contraceptive protection and will not become pregnant. To effectively prevent pregnancy, it is often necessary to use a birth control pill with a higher estrogen content, and it may be wise to add another method of contraception such as a barrier device (diaphragm or condom) with spermicide. Similarly, birth control pills with a low estrogen content may not be effective when taken for a gynecologic disorder such as endometriosis. Clobazam, felbamate, gabapentin, lamotrigine, levetiracetam, valproate, and vigabatrin do not interact significantly with birth control pills. However, felbamate and valproate may increase hormone levels, and a lower dose of birth control medication may be needed.

AEDs and Alcohol

Doctors and pharmacists warn patients with epilepsy not to use alcohol or to limit its use, so they are less likely than others to use or abuse it. Alcohol does not seriously alter the effectiveness of AEDs, but it can alter the blood levels of some of them. For example, moderate or large alcohol consumption in a short period can increase blood phenytoin levels. Prolonged use of alcohol can decrease blood levels of phenobarbital and phenytoin by increasing metabolism.

People who drink alcoholic beverages while taking AEDs may become intoxicated quickly. Many of these drugs have dose-related adverse effects similar to the effects of alcohol, including slurred speech, unsteadiness, dizziness, and tiredness. These effects can be especially dangerous when someone who takes AEDs has several drinks, becomes intoxicated, and has to drive, supervise small children, or operate dangerous equipment. Another danger occurs when someone taking high doses of phenobarbital or primidone drinks a very large amount of alcohol quickly. In this case, the person could lapse into a coma or die.

Persons with epilepsy should not consume more than two alcoholic beverages per 24 hours. Drinking more than this can be followed by withdrawal (most likely to occur 4–48 hours after drinking), during which time seizures are more likely to occur. Drinking more than two alcoholic beverages also is often associated with missing doses of AEDs and sleep deprivation. The combination of multiple risk factors for seizures—missed doses, alcohol withdrawal, and sleep deprivation—can provoke unusually intense or prolonged seizures.

Reducing the Cost of AEDs

Is It a Good Idea to Use Generic Drugs?

Brand-name drugs are manufactured by major pharmaceutical companies and are more expensive than generic drugs. Although generic drugs may be manufactured by large pharmaceutical companies, they are often made by smaller companies, and it may be difficult to find out who manufactures the drugs distributed by a specific pharmacy. More AEDs are now available in gneric form, and their use is also increasing because they are less expensive. For AEDs, however, the generics may not be equivalent to the brand-name preparations. The major difference between generic and brand-name medication is not the quality of the drug itself, but rather the consistency in the amount of medication and the way in which it is made. The manufacturing process can affect how much of the drug is absorbed and the rate at which it is absorbed. The absorption of generic AEDs may be more variable than for brand-name drugs. For some patients, therefore, using generic drugs is associated with fluctuating blood drug levels, leading to a potential increase in seizure frequency (low levels) and an increase in side effects (high levels).

Although there are some good, reliable generic drug products, it is often difficult to know exactly which manufacturer makes the generic drug that a person receives. The FDA requires that the bioavailability of generics must be within 20% of brand name medications. They may be lower or higher. They may vary from batch to batch for a given manufacturer and especially between manufacturers. Pharmacy suppliers often buy from different companies based on cost and availability. Thus, one generic manufacturer may have pills that are 18% over but the next one makes pills that are 19% under—this would be a 37% change in dosage despite the patient taking the "exact same dose"! Because of these unpredictable situations, most neurologists recommend brand-name epilepsy drugs only and, if generics areused, to avoid switching between different manufacturers' products.

The change from a brand-name drug to a generic drug should only be made with the doctor's approval. Prescriptions have a box for "DAW" (Dispense as Written). If the doctor writes a brand name and does not check this box (or write DAW inside it), the pharmacist can substitute a generic drug. If a brand-name drug is indicated, the patient may be responsible to pay the difference between the cost of the brand name and generic (which can a difference of more than $250/month for one drug). Many patients cannot afford brand name AEDs and must use generics. If a generic drug is substituted for a brand-name drug, the pharmacist should notify the patient and the doctor so that any additional tests that may be required can be ordered. Patients should always check their AEDs before leaving the pharmacy and question the pharmacist if the pills look different.

Other Ways to Cut Costs

AEDs are expensive, but there are several ways to cut their costs. Larger dose forms of drugs often cost the same, or are only slightly more expensive than lower doses. Therefore, as an example, if you need to take 100 mg of medication, it is often much cheaper to have the doctor prescribe 200 mg pills and take half a pill. Not all pills can be cut, though, so check with the doctor. When choosing health insurance, find out if there is a prescription plan and, if so, how the plan works. Compare the possible increased costs of a health care plan that includes partial or complete coverage for medications to the costs of the drugs, as well as the other benefits.

Before purchasing medication, shop around. There may be considerable price differences between pharmacies. Large pharmacies, chain stores, mail-order, and Internet plans frequently offer lower prices (Appendix D), and some pharmacies offer discounts if you purchase larger quantities. Pharmacy services can also help. For example, membership in the Epilepsy Foundation includes access to the AARP pharmacy. Most major manufacturers of brand-name AEDs offer a program to make drugs available to patients with limited incomes (www.epilepsy.com/epilepsy/drugassist_links.html; see Appendix D).

Discontinuing AEDs

Getting off AEDs is the goal of most people with well-controlled seizures. Chapter 17 discusses the way most children "outgrow" epilepsy and are able to stop their drug therapy. These principles apply to most adults. If someone has had only one seizure and is seizure-free for 6-12 months, many doctors will consider discontinuing the medication. For patients with recurrent seizures, most doctors consider discontinuing

AEDs after a seizure-free period of 1–4 years. Good prognostic factors for coming off medications and staying seizure-free include (1) few seizures before taking AEDs, (2) seizures were easily controlled with one drug, and (3) normal results on the neurologic examination, MRI, and EEG.

For certain types of seizures, such as benign rolandic epilepsy, it can be predicted with a high degree of certainty that seizures will not recur after age 16 even if medication is discontinued. By contrast, the seizures in juvenile myoclonic epilepsy are often well controlled, but seizures are likely to return if the medication is stopped.

12 | Drugs Used to Treat Epilepsy

D rug selection is a complicated clinical decision, influenced by data from controlled trials, the doctor's experience and bias, and the patient and family input. Factors that should be considered include the seizure type and epilepsy syndrome, likely effectiveness and possible side effects, cost, how often it must be taken, and interactions. This chapter reviews the most frequently used AEDs and some experimental ones; the characteristics and side effects are summarized in Tables 12.1 and 12.2. Appendix C lists the major interactions that these drugs have with other medications.

How does my medication work?

AEDs help restore balance to the brain's electrical activity. Simplistically, seizures can be considered the result of too much "positive activity" (excitation) or too little "negative activity" (inhibition) at the level of individual nerve cells and networks of nerve cells. Most AEDs work through a variety of ways to either reduce the excess or increase inhibition (Table 12.3). For example, many AEDs influenece ion channels, which regulate how much of an electrically charged ion (e.g., sodium, calcium, or potassium) can get into a nerve cell. Others alter levels of chemical neurotransmitters that modify electrical activity.

Table 12.1. Characteristics of Antiepileptic Drugs When Used Alone

Drug	Average daily dose (mg) for adults	Average daily dose (mg/kg) for children*	Time to peak blood level[a] (hr)	Therapeutic blood levels (µg/ ml blood)	Half-life[b] (hr)
Acetazolamide	250–1000		2–4	10–30	10–12
Carbamazepine[c]	800–1400	<6 y-o: 15–35 6–12 y-o: <1000	2–12	5–12	6–22
Clonazepam[d]	0.5–10	0.1–0.2	1–4	20–80 (ng/ml)	15–50
Clorazepate	3.75–22.5	3.75–15 mg	0.5–2		30–100
Ethosuximide[d]	500–1500	3–6 y-o: 20–30 >6 y-o: 500–1000	1–4	50–100	25–70
Felbamate[d]	1400–3600		1–4	30–100	14–20
Gabapentin[d]	900–3600	25–50	2–4	4–16	5–7
Lamotrigine[d]	200–500 (less with VPA and more with enzyme inducers)	2–8	2–4	2–14	7–60[g]
Levetiracetam	750–3000	10–40	1–2	15–55	6–8
Oxcarbazepine	600–2400	6–50	3–6	10–35**	10
Phenobarbital	90–180	2–8	2–12	12–40	26–140
Phenytoin	300–600	4–7	4–8	10–20	14–30[b]
Primidone	250–500	<25	2–5	5–18	12
Tiagabine	32–56	0.5–2		5–70 mg/ml	4–9

(Continued)

Table 12.1. (Continued)					
Topiramate	200–400	3–9		2–25	20
Valproate[c]	1000–3000	15–60	2–8 1–3[i]	50–120	8–15
Zonisamide	100–600	2–12	5–6	10–40	40–60

* Actual doses use can vary considerably, as some patients may be seizure-free at lower doses and others may require and tolerate higher doses. When used in combination with other drugs, dosages may vary.
** MHD, active metabolite, is measured.
[a] After blood drug levels reach steady state; may reflect sustained release preparation.
[b] Children metabolize many drugs more rapidly than adults do, so the half-life is often shorter in children.
[c] Active metabolite.
[d] In general, when these drugs are given together with carbamazepine, phenobarbital, phenytoin, or primidone, their blood level is lower and their half-life is shorter.
[g] Valproate prolongs the half-life of lamotrigine.
[h] The half-life of phenytoin increases as the dose or blood level increase.
[i] After oral dose of valproate.

My doctor recommended a drug but it is not FDA approved for monotherapy.

The U.S. Food and Drug Administration (FDA) requires specific study designs for a drug to receive an indication. There are three main areas in epilepsy where doctors prescribe beyond FDA indications: pediatrics, generalized epilepsy, and monotherapy.

Pediatrics and Generalized Epilepsy: Most drugs are studied mainly, or exclusively, in adults with partial epilepsy. Drugs that are effective for adults with partial epilepsy have proven effective for children with partial epilepsy. However, children can have different drug metabolism and side effect profiles than adults.

The leap from adults to children with partial epilepsy is much smaller than from partial epilepsy to generalized epilepsy. Some drugs for partial epilepsy can make generalized seizure types worse (Table 11.1). However, other drugs approved initially for partial epilepsy are now proven effective for generalized epilepsy (lamotrigine, levetiracetam, topiramate). Others, such as levetiracetam, felbamate, and zonisamide, also appear effective in many patients with generalized epilepsy, although they do not have an FDA indication for this disorder.

Monotherapy: A drug must be proven to be more effective than placebo to receive a monotherapy indication. Equivalence to an established,

Table 12.2. Side Effects of Antiepileptic Drugs

Drug	Dose-related side effects	Rare idiosyncratic side effects	Long-term side effects
Acetazolamide	Increased frequency of urination, tingling of face, fingers, toes	Kidney stones	None
Benzodiazepines Clobazam Clonazepam Clorazepate Diazepam Lorazepam	Tiredness, dizziness, unsteadiness, impaired attention and memory, hyperactivity, depression, irritability, aggressivity, drooling (children), nausea, loss of appetite	Extremely rare–low platelets or blood cells	None
Carbamazepine and oxcarbazepine	Nausea, vomiting, blurred or double vision, tiredness, dizziness, unsteadiness, impotence memory problems, slurred speech, low sodium (hyponatremia), tremor, weight gain, rash or fever[b]	Very low blood cell counts (bone marrow suppression) liver damage, severe rash, hypersensitivity reaction, heart block (a blockage of electrical impulses in the heart)	Bone loss
Ethosuximide	Nausea and vomiting, loss of appetite, weight loss, behavioral changes, tiredness, dizziness, earache	Very low blood cell counts (bone marrow suppression)	None
Felbamate	Headache, insomnia, irritability, nausea, vomiting, weight loss	Bone marrow or liver failure (combined risk estimated at about 1 in 4500); rash, severe rash	None
Gabapentin	Dizziness, tiredness, weight gain, leg swelling	None	None
Lamotrigine	Insomnia, nausea, unsteadiness blurred/ double vision	Severe rash	None

(Continued)

Table 12.2. (Continued)			
Levetira-cetam	Tiredness, dizziness, unsteadiness, irritability	Unknown	Unknown
Phenobarbital, mephobarbital, and primidone	Tiredness, depression, hyperactivity, dizziness, memory problems, impotence, slurred speech, nausea, anemia, rash[b] or fever, low calcium levels and bone loss	Liver damage, severe rash, hypersensitivity reaction	Bone loss, soft tissue growths, rheumatological disorders (frozen shoulder, stiffening of fingers)
Phenytoin	Tiredness, dizziness, memory problems, rash[b] or fever, gum overgrowth, growth of facial hair, anemia, acne, slurred speech, low calcium and bone loss	Liver damage, severe rash and other hypersensitivity reactions, behavioral changes	Bone loss, nerve damage, possible damage to cerebellum (part of brain)
Tiagabine	Dizziness, tiredness, mood changes	Status epilepticus	None
Topiramate	Dizziness, tiredness, decreased appetite, impaired concentration and word finding, memory problems, mood changes	Kidney stones, rash, glaucoma, heat stroke (in children)	None
Valproate	Nausea and vomiting, tiredness, weight gain, hair loss, tremor	Liver damage, very low platelet counts, pancreatic inflammation, hearing loss, behavioral changes	Bone loss, hair loss, hair texture change, weight gain
Vigabatrin	Tiredness, weight gain	None	Damage to retina and impairment of peripheral vision
Zonisamide	Drowsiness, dizziness, loss of appetite, GI discomfort	Kidney stones, rash	Possible bone loss

WBC, white blood cell count; CBC, complete blood cell count; GI, gastrointestinal.
[a] Some of the side effects (very low blood cell or platelet count, liver damage, hypersensitivity reactions, severe rash, pancreatic inflammation) are serious and potentially fatal.
[b] Rash and fever are common (3–6% of patients) but not related to the dosage.

Table 12.3. Mechanisms of Antiepileptic Drug Action

Decrease Excitation (Reduce the Excessive Electrical Activity)

Decrease Flow in Sodium Channels

> carbamazepine, felbamate, lamotrigine, oxcarbazepine, phenobarbital, phenytoin, topiramate, valproate, zonisamide

Decrease Flow in Calcium Channels

> ethosuximide, gabapentin, pregabalin, zonisamide

Decrease Flow in Potassium Channels

> levetiracetam

Decrease Action of Excitatory Neurotransmitter Glutamate

> felbamate, lamotrigine, topiramate

Increase Inhibition

Increase Action of Brain's Inhibitory Neurotransmitter GABA

> benzodiazepines, felbamate, phenobarbital, tiagabine, topiramate, valproate, vigabatrin

Uncertain Effects

Binding to Synaptic Vesicle Protein

> Levetiracetam

effective AED will not satisfy the FDA (although appeals are ongoing). This is a problem. Patients who volunteer for drug studies are usually those with very difficult-to-control partial seizures. New-onset and well-controlled patients rarely volunteer for drug studies. It is dangerous and unethical to take someone who has seizures on effective medications and randomize them to either a new drug (which may not be effective) or placebo. So most new drugs are tested in "add-on" or adjunctive studies: patients on an existing drug therapy are randomized to receive the new drug or placebo. Such studies can provide an adjunctive ("add-on") but not a monotherapy indication for partial epilepsy. These challenges, as well as expense, lead many companies to settle for the adjunctive indication, knowing that many doctors (like me) will prescribe the AED as monotherapy based on the clinical situation.

FDA indications are a conservative guide to prescribing AEDs, but one that may not serve patients' best interests. If a drug is effective and well tolerated, but only indicated in adults as adjunctive therapy, many epilepsy experts will use it in children or as monotherapy. More caution is needed in using a drug approved only in partial epilepsy for those with generalized epilepsy. However, if other medications are ineffective or intolerable, and clinical data strongly suggest effectiveness, a trial may be worthwhile. Regardless of the specific therapy, the patient and doctor must jointly assess beneficial and detrimental effects-for even those used within an FDA indication may be ineffective or occasionally exacerbate seizures.

How do you know if they are safe to take for a long time?

Doctors have much more long-term safety information about drugs such as carbamazepine, phenytoin, and valproate than about the medications approved after 1995. Although safety screens and monitoring are better now, significant problems can still occur. The relatively high and very serious risk of liver or bone marrow failure associated with felbamate were identified a year after FDA approval. In contrast, the hormonal side effects of valproate were first reported nearly 20 years after FDA approval. And although the increased risk of birth defects with valproate was recognized within a decade of its approval, the neurodevelopmental effects on children whose mothers took valproate during pregnancy was not recognized for nearly three decades.

Doctors cannot state with certainty that no new side effects will be identified after long-term use of new AEDs. The overall safety profile of the new drugs appears more favorable than most older drugs, especially regarding long-term effects. For example, gabapentin, lamotrigine, and levetiracetam do not cause bone loss, and none of the new drugs cause the peripheral nerve damage or soft-tissue changes associated with phenytoin or phenobarbital. Also, with additional data, some dangers appear smaller. The risk of bone marrow failure appeared high with carbamazepine after it was initially introduced, but better data reveals it is extremely low (-1/50,000). One study found a nearly 1/50 risk of life-threatening rash in children treated with lamotrigine, but started and increased slowly, the risks may be closer to 1/10,000. The risks and benefits of any new therapy must be balanced. For example, is a 35%

reduction in seizure frequency worth the possible additional side effects, inconvenience, and cost of a second drug?

Drugs Commonly Used Against Epilepsy

The following pages discuss the most commonly used AEDs, listed alphabetically. A discussion of the role of benzodiazepines (clonazepam, clobazam, clorazepate, diazepam, lorazepam) follows (see page 149–151).

Acetazolamide

Acetazolamide (Diamox®) can be used with another drug to treat absence and myoclonic seizures. It is also used to treat partial or generalized seizures that occur more often around the time of menstruation (catamenial epilepsy; see Chapter 7). Acetazolamide inhibits the enzyme carbonic anhydrase. Proof of its long-term effectiveness in epilepsy is limited. The drug can become less effective over time (tolerance). Common side effects include dizziness, tingling of the lips, fingertips, and toes, and increased urination (it is a mild diuretic). About 1–2% of patients taking it develop kidney stones, so patients should drink plenty of fluids, especially in hot environments. Since the ketogenic diet (see Chapter 14), topiramate, and zonisamide can also predispose to kidney stones, acetazolamide should be used cautiously with these therapies.

Acetazolamide is available in 125- and 250-mg tablets. There is no clearly defined therapeutic range of blood drug levels. Acetazolamide is also used to treat altitude sickness.

Carbamazepine

Carbamazepine (Tegretol®, Tegretol-XR®, Carbatrol®) is a first-line drug for all types of partial seizures and partial epilepsy syndromes (except benign rolandic epilepsy, in which it may increase seizure activity). The liver metabolizes it more rapidly after taking it for several weeks (i.e., *autoinduction*). Therefore, a carbamazepine level measured 8–12 weeks after the start of therapy is often lower than a level measured after 2 weeks.

Common side effects include tiredness, blurred or double vision, nausea, dizziness, or unsteadiness. It may slightly reduce attention and the speed of thinking. Rash occurs in 5–7% of patients. During the first month of treatment, avoid heavy sunlight exposure, which may increase the risk of rash. Decreased vitamin D levels and bone loss may follow long-term use. Very rare (<1/25,000) life-threatening side effects are liver or bone marrow failure. Carbamazepine can lower the amount of sodium (salt) in the blood. It may cause mild weight gain (usually less than 15 pounds in an adult).

Carbamazepine is available as a generic drug in various strengths. Tegretol is available as a chewable 100- and 200-mg tablet. Tegretol elixir is a liquid that contains 100 mg of the drug in each 5 ml (about 1 teaspoon). Tegretol-XR (extended release) is available in round tablets: 100 mg (yellow), 200 mg (pink), and 400 mg (beige). The shell of the pill, which is not absorbed, has a small hole in it, which slowly releases the medication. There is no need to worry if the shell is found in the stool; the medicine has been absorbed. Tegretol-XR pills pass through some children too rapidly for all of the medication to be absorbed, however. Carbatrol is another sustained-release form in 100 mg (light blue), 200 mg (gray and turquoise) and 300 mg (black and turquoise) capsules. Off-label (non-FDA) uses include stabilization of mood in patients with bipolar disorder and neuropathic pain (pain due to nerve, spinal cord, or brain disorders).

Ethosuximide

Ethosuximide (Zarontin®) is used to treat only absence seizures. It has no effect against (or may even worsen) myoclonic, tonic-clonic, or partial seizures. Side effects include nausea and vomiting, loss of appetite, weight loss, behavioral changes, tiredness, and dizziness. Ethosuximide is available as a 250-mg gelcap (amber).

Felbamate

Felbamate (Felbatol®) is effective in treating partial and secondarily generalized tonic-clonic seizures and Lennox-Gastaut syndrome and may also help control primary generalized seizures. The drug is usually given two to three times daily. It is generally well tolerated, and many patients report feeling "more awake" and "brighter" on it. Common side effects are decreased appetite, weight loss, insomnia, and headache. Cognitive and behavioral problems are uncommon and are usually mild.

Many adults can tolerate doses of 2000–3600 mg per day. Felbamate is available as an elixir (600 mg per 5 ml [teaspoon]; fruit punch flavor) and in 400-mg (yellow) and 600-mg (peach) tablets.

Felbamate had a ~1 in 4000 risk of bone marrow failure or liver failure that was fatal in ~1 in 3 of affected individuals (~1 in 12,000 died) before blood tests were carefully monitored. Its use is now strictly limited to patients in whom the benefits outweigh the risks. Blood cell counts and liver function tests should be performed often (every 2 weeks is recommended), at least during the first year of therapy, when most of these serious problems occur. These tests can provide an early warning of danger and can lower but not eliminate the risks. Felbamate can also produce rash, which can rarely take a serious form that is life-threatening (Stevens Johnson syndrome/toxic epidermal necrolysis).

Gabapentin

Gabapentin (Neurontin®) is effective for all partial seizures, but it is not effective for any primary generalized seizures. Approved for adjunctive use, it can be effective in monotherapy for some patients. Gabapentin is beneficial for some pain syndromes. It is an amino acid that is chemically related to the inhibitory neurotransmitter, GABA. It has a short half-life (~6 hours) and usually needs to be taken three times a day.

Gabapentin is usually very well tolerated; the most common side effects are dose-related tiredness and dizziness, which often improve after several weeks. Other side effects include headache, unsteadiness, visual changes, abdominal discomfort, edema (swelling) in the limbs (especially feet), and weight gain. Behavioral problems such as irritability and hyperactivity can occur in children. Gabapentin may improve mood and emotional well-being. Gabapentin does not cause life-threatening side effects. Most adults take 1200–3600 mg/day.

Gabapentin is considered less effective in controlling partial seizures than some other drugs. Initial trials were done with a maximum dose of 1800 mg/day, and now higher doses are commonly used. At 3600 mg/day, approximately 40% (1440 mg) of the drug is absorbed. However, if a person takes 4800 mg/day, only about 33% is absorbed (~1585 mg), limiting the theoretical benefits of very high doses. Gabapentin is excreted unchanged in the urine. The lack of liver metabolism and protein binding means that it does not interact with other drugs.

Gabapentin is available as a generic (capsule and tablet) and as brand-name Neurontin in hard gelatin capsules with doses of 100 mg (white), 300 mg (yellow), 400 mg (orange), and 600 and 800 mg (white ovals) scored tablets. An elixir (250 mg/5 cc) is also available.

Lamotrigine

Lamotrigine (Lamictal®) is approved for the treatment of all partial seizures, primary generalized tonic-clonic seizures, and Lennox-Gastaut syndrome. It is also effective in treating absence seizures. It can be used alone as a monotherapy or as an adjunctive therapy. Its approximately 24-hour half-life is affected by other AEDs: roughly doubled by valproate and halved by drugs that induce liver enzymes (e.g., carbamazepine, phenytoin). Lamotrigine levels may be decreased by acetaminophen (Tylenol®) and contraceptive pills and patches. Lamotrigine is usually given once or twice a day (especially in patients taking drugs that induce liver enzymes), adult dosages range from 150 to 600 mg per day.

Lamotrigine is generally well tolerated; for some patients, energy, mood, and emotional well-being improve. Side effects include dizziness, unsteadiness, blurred vision, headache, nausea, diarrhea, unsteadiness, insomnia, tiredness, and rash. The frequency and severity of rash are greater if the dosage is increased rapidly. The rash most usually involves the trunk, arms, or face and is more likely if patients also take valproate. A potentially life-threatening rash (Stevens-Johnson syndrome) can develop, especially in children on valproate in whom the dose is increased rapidly. Lamotrigine should be started at a very low dosage and increased very gradually, especially if the patient is taking valproate. This slow titration is a disadvantage, as it can take 1–2 months to obtain a therapeutic effect.

Lamisil®—an antifungal drug—has been mistakenly given instead of Lamictal, so always read the label!

Lamotrigine is available as white chewable tablets that are 2-mg, 5-mg, or 25-mg; also as 100-mg (peach), 150-mg (cream), and 200-mg (blue) tablets. There are currently no capsules or liquids available. Generic form is available.

Levetiracetam

Levetiracetam (Keppra®) is FDA approved as adjunctive therapy for children and adults with partial epilepsy as well as treatment of myoclonic seizures in patients with juvenile myocolonic epilepsy and primary generalized tonic-clonic seizures. The half-life is 7–12 hours. The drug is mainly excreted unchanged in the urine; there is no liver metabolism and no known interactions with other drugs. The most commonly reported side effect is tiredness. Uncommon side effects include dizziness, nausea, unsteadiness, weakness, headache, and behavioral changes. Irritability and depression are the most common side effects that lead to discontinuation. These problems are more common with rapid dosage increases, in children, and in patients with developmental disabilities. Rash is very rare. The adult dosage is usually 1000–3000 mg/day, given in two or occasionally three doses.

Levetiracetam is available as Keppra® tablets, which are oblong and coated with a film. Doses are 250 mg (blue), 500 mg (yellow), 750 mg (orange), and 1000 mg (white). This drug is also available as an elixir (100 mg/ml) and for intravenous use. No generic is available.

Oxcarbazepine

Oxcarbazepine (Trileptal®) is closely related chemically to carbamazepine. It is FDA approved as monotherapy and adjunctive therapy to treat partial seizures in children and adults. Its side effect profile is similar to carbamazepine: tiredness, dizziness, headache, blurred or double vision, and unsteadiness. Among patients in whom carbamazepine caused a rash, about 25% will have a rash when later treated with oxcarbazepine. It has few cognitive side effects. The level of sodium in the blood may become low (hyponatremia), which may cause tiredness and dizziness and increase seizure frequency. Decreased vitamin D levels and bone loss may follow long-term use.

The half-life is about 2 hours, but its antiseizure effect is due to the formation of an active byproduct (monohydroxyderivative, MHD) with a half-life of 10 hours. Oxcarbazepine is available as Trileptal in three sizes of oblong, scored, mustard-yellow tablets—150, 300, and 600 mg—and as an oral suspension (300 mg/5 ml). No generic is available.

Phenytoin

Phenytoin (Dilantin®, Phenytek®) is a first-line drug for all types of partial seizures. Adult dosages range from 200 to 600 mg per day. In emergency settings, it (or its prodrug fosphenytoin [Cerebyx®]) may be given intravenously to achieve therapeutic levels rapidly. Its long half-life (16–28 hours) allows it to be taken once or twice a day. The half-life may be under 12 hours in children or patients taking low doses (the higher the dose, the longer the half-life). Once-a-day dosing is not advised for these patients because the trough (lowest) blood levels of the drug may be very low, increasing the risk of seizures.

Side effects include tiredness, dizziness, unsteadiness, slurred speech, acne, rash (~6% of patients, rarely serious or life-threatening), and darker or excessive hair (hirsutism), most troublesome for girls and women. Cognitive and behavioral problems are infrequent and usually mild at therapeutic blood levels. Long-term use can lower vitamin D levels and cause bone loss, soft-tissue growths, and, rarely, nerve injury (neuropathy) or loss of tissue in the cerebellum of the brain (possibly related to very high blood levels). Because phenytoin can cause gum overgrowth (hyperplasia), maintaining regular dental visits and flossing are important. Very rare (<1/100,000) life-threatening side effects include liver failure and bone marrow failure (aplastic anemia).

The metabolism and clearance of phenytoin slows as the dose rises. This can cause very slow accumulation and overdose, which can lead to hospitalization. The amount in the bloodstream can continue to increase for up to a month after a dose change. Conversely, reduction in the dose may lead to unusually large decreases in the blood level that can lead to increased seizure activity.

Phenytoin is available as a generic 100-mg capsule. Dilantin is available as a 30-mg capsule (white with pink stripe) or a 100-mg capsule (white with a red stripe) or as a 50-mg chewable tablet (Infatab). Phenytek is available as a 200- and 300-mg capsule. Dilantin is also available as an elixir (liquid) and as an intravenous preparation, which should only be used in the hospital. Intravenous fosphenytoin (Cerebyx) is safer because it does not cause serious complications if it leaks out of the vein. Fosphenytoin is a rapidly converted into phenytoin by the liver.

Pregabalin

Pregabalin (Lyrica®) is approved as an adjunctive therapy for adults with partial epilepsy. It is closely related to gabapentin and is also an analogue of GABA that has efficacy in neuropathic pain and anxiety disorders. Common side effects include tiredness and dizziness. Other side effects include tremor, unsteadiness, visual changes, dry mouth, and peripheral (mainly feet) edema (swelling). Weight gain can occur with long-term use. There are no known life-threatening side effects.

The half-life is 8–10 hours; it is usually dosed twice a day. It is excreted unchanged in the urine and has no drug interactions. Adult doses range from 150 to 600 mg per day. It comes in 25-, 50-, 75-, 100-, 150-, 200-, and 300-mg tablets. No generic is available.

Tiagabine

Tiagabine (Gabitril®) is FDA approved for treating partial epilepsy in patients age 12 years and older. It prolongs the action of GABA by blocking its reuptake by cells. The half-life is approximately 5–8 hours. Twice-a-day dosing is effective. However, tiagabine is often given three times a day. The dose is often started at 4–10 mg/day and increased gradually to 32–56 mg/day.

Common side effects include dizziness, tiredness, nervousness, and headache. Occasional side effects are tremor, nausea, diarrhea, weakness, irritability, difficulty concentrating, or confusion. Rarely, continuous seizures (status epilepticus) have occurred. For some patients, tiagabine improves mood. Drug interactions are uncommon, although tiagabine is metabolized more rapidly in patients taking drugs that induce liver enzymes.

Tiagabine is available as 4-mg (yellow round), 12-mg (green oval), 16-mg (blue oval), and 20-mg (pink oval) tablets. No capsules or liquids are currently available, nor is there a generic form.

Topiramate

Topiramate (Topamax®) is approved to for monotherapy and adjunctive therapy in patients 10 years or older with partial epilepsy or primary generalized tonic-clonic seizures and in patients with Lennox-Gastaut syndrome. The half-life is approximately 21 hours; it is usually given twice a day. The average daily adult dose ranges from 150 to 600 mg. Topiramate has few significant drug interactions. It can slightly raise phenytoin levels, and drugs that induce liver enzymes (e.g., carbamazepine, phenytoin) can lower topiramate levels by up to 50%.

Side effects include tiredness, dizziness, unsteadiness, weight loss, constipation, tingling (usually in the fingers, toes, or around the mouth), double vision or other visual problems, problems with concentration, slowing of thought processes, word-finding problems, depression, or irritability. Most patients tolerate the drug well when started at a low dose (25–50 mg/day) and increased slowly (25 mg/week). Because topiramate can cause kidney stones in 1–2% of patients, it should be used cautiously in patients on the ketogenic diet or taking acetazolamide or zonisamide. Patients should drink adequate fluids, especially in hot environments. It can rarely cause glaucoma and, in children, a lack of sweating that can lead to heat stroke in hot weather.

Topiramate is available as a 25-mg (white), 100-mg (yellow), and 200-mg (salmon) tablet. The tablets are not scored and as a rule should not be broken because of the bitter taste. Topiramate is also available as a 15- and 25-mg sprinkle capsule. No liquid form or generic form is available.

Valproate

Valproate (valproic acid; Depakene®, Depakote® [divalproex sodium]) is effective in treating all generalized and partial seizure types. It is a first-line drug for several primary generalized epilepsy syndromes (juvenile myoclonic epilepsy and absence epilepsy with tonic-clonic seizures). Valproate is also an effective preventive therapy when taken every day for migraine headaches and bipolar disorder.

Common side effects of valproate—weight gain and tremor—limit its use. Additionally, side effects on hormonal function (e.g., irregular menses, polycystic ovarian syndrome) as well as birth defects and developmental delays in children born to mothers on valproate further limit its use in women of childbearing age. Other side effects include tiredness, dizziness, nausea, vomiting, hair loss, and behavioral changes such as depression in adults and irritability in children. Long-term use of valproate can cause bone loss and ankle swelling. Rare and dangerous side effects include liver damage, very low numbers of platelets (clotting cells), inflammation of the pancreas, confusion, and hearing loss.

Hair loss and pancreatic inflammation may be prevented or reduced by taking the minerals selenium (10–20 µg/day) and zinc (25–50 mg/day), although proof is lacking; many high-potency multivitamins contain these mineral dosages. The risk of life-threatening liver toxicity is very low: approximately 1 in 30,000 adults and children over 2 years of age who are taking the drug. The highest risk (~1/500 is in children under age 6 months on at least one other AED).

Valproate is available as a generic drug in 125-, 250-, and 500-mg tablets. Depakene (valproate) is available as a 250-mg tablet (red). It is also available in liquid form. A delayed-release preparation, divalproex sodium (Depakote), is available as a 125-mg sprinkle capsule and as 125-mg (red), 250-mg (light orange), and 500-mg (pink) tablets; and an extended release form, Depakote ER® (white, 250-mg tablet; a gray, 500-mg tablet).

Vigabatrin

Vigabatrin (Sabril®) is used mainly to treat infantile spasms and medically refractory partial seizures. Vigabatrin is marketed in many countries, but not the United States, although it can be legally obtained. Its half-life is 5–6 hours, but its action lasts 6 days due to its effect. It is usually taken twice a day.

Vigabatrin typically is well tolerated. Drowsiness and fatigue are the most common side effects. Others include irritability and nervousness, dizziness, headache, depression, and rarely, psychosis. Unfortunately, as many as 30% of patients taking vigabatrin develop potentially irreversible retinal damage that impairs the peripheral field of vision. This safety issue prevented FDA approval and limits its use almost exclusively to patients with infantile spasms or patients with tuberous sclerosis and partial epielpsy. Vigabatrin is available as a 500-mg white oval tablet and 500-mg sachets.

Zonisamide

Zonisamide (Zonegran®) is a sulfonamide drug used to treat partial seizures but with evidence that it may be effective for primary generalized absence, myoclonic, and tonic-clonic seizures. It is slowly but completely absorbed over 3–6 hours and is more than 90% metabolized in the liver. The half-life is 40–60 hours.

Side effects include drowsiness, dizziness, unsteadiness, decreased appetite/weight loss, stomach discomfort, irritability, headache, mild cognitive problems, and rash. Kidney stones occur in 1–2% of patients. Children may have decreased sweating, which can lead to heat stroke. Zonisamide should generally not be used by patients taking acetazolamide and topiramate (which also cause kidney stones). Patients should drink adequate fluids, especially in hot environments. Zonegran is available as a 25-, 50-, and 100-mg capsule; there is no liquid, sprinkle or intravenous form. Generic 25-, 50-, and 100 mg capsules are available.

The Role of Benzodiazepines in Treating Epilepsy

Benzodiazepines (clonazepam, clobazam, clorazepate, diazepam, lorazepam) are effective as short-term therapy to help prevent or stop generalized and partial seizures. They are also used to treat anxiety. Tolerance often develops within weeks, however, so that the same dose of medication has less effect, whether for epilepsy or anxiety.

Benzodiazepines are very commonly used to stop prolonged or repetitive seizures. Intravenous forms are available in the hospital. Rectal, buccal (between gum and lip), or sublingual (under the tongue) benzodiazepines can be used outside the hospital. Benzodiazepines are sometimes used to stop a cluster of seizures (e.g., a person who, once a month, has one complex partial seizure in the morning followed by several that day). A person who has a characteristic warning that lasts at least 15 minutes before seizures may prevent the larger seizure by taking a benzodiazepine when the warning begins. Long-term benzodiazepine therapy for epilepsy remains controversial, although certain benzodiazepines can be effective (see below).

Benzodiazepine side effects include cause tiredness, dizziness, unsteadiness, irritability, hyperactivity (in children), drooling (in children), depression (usually in adults), nausea, and loss of appetite. They cause more cognitive problems than most other AEDs. One danger is the tendency to increase the dose as tolerance develops. Side effects may outpace benefits. Moreover, gradual increases over months or years can lead to personality changes (irritability, depression, or decreased motivation) or cognitive problems (impaired memory) that go unnoticed or are attributed to "epilepsy" or "constitution." This is especially common for individuals with developmental disabilities, often worsening cognitive function and quality of life.

For epilepsy patients, seizures may become more frequent or more severe if the benzodiazepine dosage is decreased or the drug is discontinued. The longer the person takes the drug and the higher the dosage, the greater the tolerance and therefore the higher the risk of worsening seizure control. Even small, gradual dose reductions can temporarily increase seizure activity, but reducing these sedating medications often brings the long-term reward of fewer side effects.

Despite these limitations, benzodiazepines can be used safely and effectively for some patients. For example, clobazam in children with partial epilepsy is comparable in side effects and seizure control to carbamazepine. In addition, for seizures that mainly occur during sleep or shortly after awakening, benzodiazepines at bedtime control seizures and improve sleep.

Clobazam

Clobazam (Frisium®, Urbanyl®) has a slightly different chemical ring structure than the other benzodiazepines, which may reduce tolerance during long-term use. Clobazam is a safe medication, approved in almost all countries except the United States. Clobazam is effective in treating partial and generalized seizures, but is most often used for partial seizures. It is used mainly as an add-on (adjunctive) drug in partial epilepsy. Its half-life is 18 hours, although an active metabolite has a half-life of 40 hours. Side effects include tiredness, unsteadiness, irritability, and mild cognitive problems. The drug should not be stopped abruptly owing to the risk of withdrawal seizures. It is produced as a 10-mg tablet or capsule.

Clonazepam

Clonazepam (Klonopin®) is used to treat absence and myoclonic seizures and can help stop seizure clusters. Clonazepam is available as a generic drug and as the brand-name Klonopin in a 0.5-mg (orange), 1.0-mg (blue), and 2.0-mg (white) round tablet.

Clorazepate

Clorazepate (Tranxene®) is used to treat partial seizures as an add-on (adjunctive) therapy. Clorazepate is available as a generic drug and as the brand-name Tranxene in scored triangular tablets: 3.75 mg (gray), 7.5 mg (yellow), and 15 mg (pink); and as Tranxene-SD® round (nonscored) tablets: 11.25 mg (purple) and 22.5 mg (tan/peach).

Diazepam

Diazepam (Valium®, Diastat®) is used to treat status epilepticus and seizure clusters. Rectal diazepam (Diastat) is given by patients' families and caregivers to treat prolonged or serial seizures. Oral diazepam can help prevent seizure clusters, but its relatively slow absorption limits its effectiveness via this route; absorption is much more rapid through the rectal route. Because it can impair breathing, however, rectal diazepam should only be given at the dose recommended by a doctor. If seizures do not diminish after the first rectal dose, a second one should be given only with a doctor's approval.

Diastat and the Diastat AcuDial are available as a preloaded syringe for rectal administration of diazepam in doses bewteen 2.5 and 20 mg. Other liquid forms of diazepam may also be given rectally (with a very small syringe).

Lorazepam

Lorazepam (Ativan®) is used to treat seizure clusters and occasionally to treat chronic epilepsy. Lorazepam can be given orally, sublingually (under the tongue), and by intramuscular and intravenous injections. It has a half-life of 8–20 hours and, like diazepam, can cause serious breathing impairment, especially when given intravenously at higher doses. Lorazepam should only be used as recommended by a physician. It is available in three sizes of white, pentagon-shaped tablets: 0.5-, 1-, and 2-mg.

Midazolam

Midazolam is a rapidly acting benzodiazepine that is used buccally (between the lip and gum) in many other countries to treat seizure clusters or prolonged seizures. Pediatric studies, using doses of 2.5–10 mg of midazolam in patients with active seizures, suggest it is equal in safety but may be more rapid in onset and more effective than rectal diazepam.

Investigational AEDs

More than a dozen AEDs are now in development; some are approved for use outside the United States. These drugs are the "pipeline" of future medical therapy. Patients with uncontrolled seizures or disabling side effects desperately need better drugs. However, new drugs can also help patients who "seem fine" with, for example, reduced risk of bone loss, sedation, weight gain, and other side effects. We need more effective and safer drugs.

New drug development remains difficult and expensive. The introduction of many new drugs has decreased the incentive of companies to
invest since the market is more saturated. Mergers have created large
pharmaceutical companies that need "billion dollar blockbusters," and
the epilepsy market is less likely to provide one than other disorders,
such as hypercholesterolemia. Bringing a new drug from the lab to the
patient is a very expensive and lengthy process. Many potential drugs
have similar mechanisms of action to existing drugs. We need drugs
with new mechanisms, since patients refractory to drugs that work
on sodium channels may be refractory to new drugs that also work on
sodium channels. Developing new models of epilepsy may be critical to
helping those with seizures resistant to current therapy. FDA regulatory
issues also limits new drug development. Since most drugs are tested
in patients with seizures that are controlled with many medications,
indications are often limited to "adjunctive" (or "add-on") use rather
than monotherapy and chronic refractory patients rather than patients
in whom seizures are of recent onset. Newer study designs are helping
to solve this problem.

Should I enroll in a drug study?

Patients with uncontrolled seizures or troublesome side effects
on available drugs may want to consider trying an experimental drug.
Those with well-controlled epilepsy and few side effects should
generally not consider enrolling in an investigational drug trial. Most
drug studies are performed at epilepsy centers. The best way of
finding out about new drug studies is to call or write nearby comprehensive epilepsy centers (see epilepsy.com or naec-epilepsy.org for a
list of centers).

Drug studies are reviewed and approved by an institutional
review board. This helps to guarantee that the risks and benefits are
carefully considered. The study must be fully explained and consent
obtained in writing from a competent adult or a parent or legal
guardian. The principal investigator in charge of the study and the
hospital's patient advocate should be available to answer any questions during the study. A patient who decides not to participate in a
study should have no fears that the doctor will be upset or with-
hold other therapies. Table 12.4 lists drugs that are currently under
investigation.

Table 12.4. Drugs Currently Under Investigation

Drug	Presumed mechanism of action
Brivaracetam	Binds SV2A
Carisbamate	Unknown (carbamate)
DP-VPA	Unknown (possibly similar to valproic acid)
Eslicarbazepine	Modifies voltage-gated sodium channel activity
Ganaxolone	Activates GABA(A) receptor complex
Lacosamide	Unknown
Retigabine	Modulates KCNQ2/3 and 3/5 potassium channel activity
Rufinamide	Unknown
Safinamide	MAO-B inhibitor, inhibits sodium and calcium channels
Seletracetam	Binds SV2A
Stiripentol	Unknown
Talampanel	Noncompetitive AMPA antagonist
Valrocemide	Unknown (possibly similar to valproic acid)

Source: Pollard JR, French J. Lancet Neurol 2006;5(12):1064–1067.

Intravenous Gamma Globulin (IVIG)

Gamma globulin is composed of antibodies derived from human blood. Antibodies help to fight bacteria and viruses. IVIG is used to bolster the immune system and treat autoimmune disorders. Its use in epilepsy patients, especially children with uncontrolled seizures, remains investigational. Although some children may improve with this therapy, many others do not.

The exception may be when an inflammatory process causes epilepsy. For example, one boy underwent unsuccessful epilepsy surgery. The brain tissue revealed a prominent inflammation, and subsequent treatment with IVIG reduced seizures more than 95%.

Gamma globulin is given as an intravenous infusion, usually in the hospital or at home under the close supervision. During the first infusion, the person must be watched closely for an allergic reaction that requires prompt treatment. Additional treatments are typically done every 2–6 weeks, usually as an outpatient. If a benefit occurs, it is usually in the first few months; the length of therapy varies.

IVIG is expensive and supply is limited. Insurance coverage and expense should be considered.

Getting Drugs Outside the United States

Some investigational drugs and other drugs (e.g., clobazam, midazolam, vigabatrin) are approved to treat epilepsy in other countries. These drugs can be imported legally into the United States with a doctor's prescription, either from foreign pharmacies by direct purchase in the country or by a mailed or faxed prescription. When the medications pass through customs (carried or mailed/delivery service), it may help to have a note from the doctor documenting epilepsy, the approval of the drug for epilepsy in another country, and the need for its use in the specific person (e.g., failure of U.S. drugs to control seizures). The supply may be limited to 3 months at one time. The drugs are usually delivered directly to the patient's home. It is essential to reorder well ahead of time since medicines may occasionally be held up at the border. Caligor Pharmacy, in New York City, can obtain some foreign epilepsy drugs but is expensive; their phone number is (212) 369–6000.

Insurance usually does not cover the costs of drugs that are not FDA approved. However, letters of appeal from both the patient and neurologist documenting the failure to respond to U.S. medications and the potential costs of alternative therapies such as surgery can help in obtaining coverage.

13 | Surgical Therapy for Epilepsy

When seizures cannot be controlled by AEDs or control can be achieved only at the cost of severe and unacceptable adverse effects, surgery may be an alternative. Pioneered in the late 1800s, the use of epilepsy surgery has dramatically risen during the past few decades, reflecting an increased awareness by both doctors and patients.

The vast majority of epilepsy surgeries are in patients with partial seizures that are difficult to control with AEDs. What is the definition of difficult-to-control seizures? The criteria have changed as the safety and effectiveness of surgery are better established. Twenty years ago, most patients who underwent epilepsy surgery had uncontrolled seizures for more than one or two decades. Surgery is now performed on patients whose seizures are uncontrolled for 1 or 2 years. A patient with an MRI showing temporal lobe scar tissue and a video EEG showing seizures arising from that area is an excellent candidate for early surgery. In general, the patient should be treated with *at least* two single drugs and with a combination of two or more drugs before surgery is considered. Medication trials must be adequate; that is, the drugs should be gradually increased to the maximally tolerated dose. The decision about how many AEDs to try depends on the individual case. For example, what are chances for success with additional medications versus surgery?

A person whose seizures persist despite three or more adequate AED trials is unlikely to achieve complete seizure control with any AED. In such cases, the risks and benefits of surgery should be carefully weighed against the costs that continued seizures and high doses that medication can impose on intellectual, psychological, social, educational, and work life. Surgery should be considered sooner rather than later.

Epilepsy surgery can be especially beneficial to persons who have seizures associated with localized structural abnormalities such as scar tissue, benign brain tumors, and blood vessels malformations (arteriovenous malformations, cavernous or venous angiomas). In the case of benign tumors and vascular malformations, removal of the abnormal tissue can successfully control the seizures. In many cases, however, especially if the seizures have occurred for years, the area adjacent to the abnormal tissue is part of the epilepsy network. Removing the abnormal tissue may or may not control of the seizures. Occasionally, the structural abnormality may have little to do with uncontrollable seizures. For example, arachnoid cysts rarely cause medically uncontrolled epilepsy. Removing the cyst is unlikely to control such seizures unless the cyst is large and exerts pressure on the brain.

Should surgery be performed sooner or later?

It is a very individual choice. Some evidence suggests that the earlier the surgery is performed, the better the outcome. Early surgery can reduce the burden of medication and seizures over many years or decades. However, patients can have epilepsy surgery after more than 30 or 40 years of uncontrolled seizures and become seizure-free. Epilepsy surgery may be a last resort for some, but if the person is a good candidate, it should be considered after several AEDs have failed.

The doctor told me the risks of doing surgery; what are the risks of not doing surgery?

Many people fail to consider the consequences of ongoing seizures and high doses of several AEDs. For some people with uncontrolled seizures, epilepsy is a progressive disorder with problems affecting memory, mood, and other functions growing worse over time. High doses of AEDs can also adversely affect mental and physical health. Together, seizures and side effects can significantly impair quality of life, including the ability to learn, to work, and to drive. There is also a more sinister risk of uncontrolled epilepsy—death. Among people whose seizures are severe enough to consider epilepsy surgery, the rate of sudden unexplained death (SUDEP; see Chapter 6) may be as high as 9 per 1000 patient years. Thus, over the course of a decade there is a 9% chance of dying from SUDEP in some patients. Compare that with the 0.1% risk of death from epilepsy surgery.

My doctor recommended surgery; do I get a second opinion? How do I decide?

The decision of whether or not to do surgery is often very difficult. Brain surgery is frightening. It is often helpful to speak to other patients. With names and numbers given out by the epilepsy center, there is the likely risk that these are folks who had great outcomes and are very pleased, not the less successful outcomes. You might ask for a number of names, but speak with other people. Internet chat rooms are helpful, but again, be wary, as it is often a select group who are actively involved.

If there is doubt about whether or not to go forward, or uncertainty about the experience of the team at one epilepsy center, seek the opinion of an epilepsy specialist outside that center. In most cases, the second opinion will make a very similar recommendation. When the two opinions disagree, try to ask each to explain their different approaches and reasons. In many cases, it is simply a different view (conservative versus aggressive) or strategy (one stage versus two stage). There is often not a "right" answer. So understanding the issues is critical to making an informed decision.

One epilepsy center said my child is not a surgical candidate; another believes that surgery can dramatically reduce but not fully control seizures.

Some epilepsy centers take a conservative approach and only recommend surgery if there is a very high likelihood that the person will become seizure-free. Others will recommend surgery as a "palliative" procedure-to reduce seizures and medication burden, although the chances for seizure freedom are small. As in other cases, the decision is ultimately about risks and benefits. If the risks are small and the benefits are moderate, it may be worth going forward. These are hard decisions that should be based on a careful consideration of the expectations with and without surgery.

Types of Surgery

There are two main types of brain surgery for epilepsy. The first, and most common, is resective surgery in which the brain area that causes seizures is removed. It is performed in cases of partial epilepsy, with or without secondarily generalized tonic-clonic seizures. Patients often imagine that the area that causes seizures is tiny—for example, the size of a pea. In almost all cases, however, the area is much larger (for example, 11/2–3 inches long and 1–11/2 inches wide). Examples of resective surgery are temporal and frontal lobectomy.

The second, less common type of epilepsy surgery is a disconnection: interrupting nerve pathways along which seizure impulses spread. Corpus callosotomy involves cutting the large fiber bundle connecting the hemispheres, but without removal of brain tissue. Functional hemispherectomy disconnects one hemisphere from the rest of the brain.

A third type of epilepsy surgery, called multiple subpial transections, can help when the seizures begin in brain areas that serve vital functions such as language, movement, or sensation. It can also help in Landau-Kleffner syndrome, an acquired language disorder in children in which frequent epilepsy waves affect the language area.

The surgically implanted vagus nerve stimulator (VNS) electrically stimulates the vagus nerve in the neck to attempt to reduce seizure activity. Investigational trials are underway to test brain stimulation to prevent seizures.

Expectations and Consequences of Epilepsy Surgery

The thought of brain surgery evokes fears and questions. Doctors, nurses, psychologists, and other patients can answer questions about the risks, complications, recovery period, and other medical details. Epilepsy surgery is major neurosurgery, and some risk is associated with it. It usually takes 4–8 weeks to resume normal activities after surgery. A patient once asked me, "Is this (epilepsy surgery) an inpatient or outpatient type of surgery?" Epilepsy surgery requires a hospital stay of 5–7 days and in some cases, 2 weeks or longer.

The procedure varies according to the type of operation. The patient is usually under general anesthesia. Occasionally, patients are kept awake while areas controlling vital functions such as language and movement are mapped with mild electrical stimulation. In such cases, a local anesthetic is used, and the surgery can be performed painlessly, since the brain is not sensitive to pain. Short-acting anesthesia allows the patient to sleep during the initial and final portions of the surgery and to be awake only during the mapping procedure.

Realistic expectations must be established before the surgery. Some persons are completely free of seizures after surgery, and many others have a marked reduction in the frequency or intensity of seizures. Some patients continue to have auras or occasional complex partial seizures. In some cases, their seizure control is not improved. After surgery, most persons who become seizure-free require AEDs, so the surgery is not a complete cure. Patients often continue to take the same medication for 6–12 months or longer after surgery. Then some can reduce and eventually come off medication.

If epilepsy can be caused by scar tissue and surgery causes scarring, can the surgery cause epilepsy?

This is an excellent question. Surgery creates a scar, but it is typically much milder than the scars that cause epilepsy. Bottom line: if all or nearly all of the epilepsy-causing tissue is successfully removed, patients usually become seizure-free.

Seizure-freedom after epilepsy surgery can be stressful for the patient or family. Seizure control may create greater pressure to work and to assume new responsibilities, and it may change relationships and other people's expectations. In addition, surgery may cause short-term memory problems or other disorders even though the seizures are fully controlled. Such problems usually improve with time. Although mood usually improves after surgery, especially in those who become seizure-free, some patients experience short-term anxiety or depression, which can be managed with supportive therapy and medications when needed.

After a period of seizure-freedom after surgery, a seizure is a huge disappointment. It can seem as though just when epilepsy is moving further into the background of one's life, it reappears. Emotionally, the recurrence of seizures can be devastating, but it does not mean that seizure control cannot be restored. In many cases, seizures are caused by missed medications, low AED blood levels caused by diarrhea or vomiting, a serious infection, sleep deprivation, excessive alcohol, or other problems. Unfortunately, some patients reduce or stop their AEDs after surgery, falsely assuming that all of the "epilepsy tissue" was removed. If side effects are bothersome, a dose reduction or change in the medication schedule can often help, but must be done under a doctor's supervision. In some patients, a single breakthrough seizure occurs for no identifiable reason. In some, intermittent seizures occur, but less frequently than before the surgery. The longer the interval of seizure freedom after surgery, the greater the chances are of never having another seizure.

Preoperative Assessment

To consider epilepsy surgery, seizures should be uncontrolled with AED doses that are tolerable. The drug trials must be adequate—that is, the seizures were not controlled despite the patient tolerating therapeutic dosages or blood levels.

How long must epilepsy be uncontrolled to consider surgery?
The answer varies. In general, most surgical patients have had seizures for at least 2 years. If the seizures are frequent, relatively short trials of medications can reveal the failure of AEDs and surgery may be considered within 6 months. If the seizures are infrequent, a longer trial is needed to determine that the therapy is ineffective. Candidates should have a good record of the AEDs that were tried, including the maximal dosages, blood levels, and side effects. When epilepsy results from a blood vessel malformation, benign tumor, or other structural lesion, fewer AED trials are needed to consider epilepsy surgery since surgery can alleviate two problems and the chances for seizure control AEDs are not very good.

If surgery is considered, studies are performed to identify the area of the brain from which the seizures arise and the areas that control vital functions such as language, memory, and movement. Hopefully, seizures do not arise from vital areas. Some areas can be removed without any changes in intellect, personality, or mood. The removal of other areas may be associated with slight deterioration or, in some cases, improvement in memory or other functions.

Noninvasive Studies

The preoperative assessment begins with a series of consultations and noninvasive tests. Noninvasive tests do not invade the body or involve surgery and, in general, involve little or no risk. The assessment includes:

- EEG recording and video-EEG monitoring to record epilepsy waves between and during seizures

- Neuroimaging by MRI (CT if that is not possible), PET, SPECT, and MEG (see Chapter 9) to identify physical or functional abnormalities in brain that help identify the area where seizures arise

- Neuropsychological studies to assess cognitive (intellectual) strengths and weaknesses, which can help to predict the area from which the seizures arise as well as possible complications of the surgery

- Assess the patient's emotional well-being and social supports by consultations with psychiatrists or psychologists, to identify problems that should be addressed before and after surgery

- Additional tests such as functional MRI or MRS (see Chapter 9) are used in some cases

Invasive Studies

The preoperative tests may also include tests that "invade" the body. Technically, insertion of a needle into a vein to draw blood is an invasive procedure, but it is so common and safe that it is not considered invasive. Invasive studies are associated with some risk, but the risk varies dramatically with the different types of tests and procedures.

Sphenoidal Electrodes

Some epilepsy centers record the EEG with sphenoidal electrodes to record brain electrical activity from deep parts of the temporal and frontal lobes. A topical anesthetic is often applied before to the skin before inserting the electrode into the cheek with a needle. The needle is immediately withdrawn, leaving in place a thin wire that is bare at the tip. The patient feels some discomfort during the insertion and for several hours afterward, particularly when yawning or chewing. The risks are minor: a small amount of bleeding, infection, or a tiny piece of the bare wire remaining in the cheek.

Subdural and Depth Electrodes

Subdural and depth electrodes record electrical activity directly from the brain and can help precisely localize the seizure focus. The decision to use subdural or depth electrodes depends on the findings from the noninvasive studies and the intracarotid sodium amobarbital test (see below). If everything points to the same area of the brain as the focus of the seizures, most epilepsy centers proceed without invasive electrodes. If the information is inconsistent or indefinite, or the focus lies in or near functional brain areas, however, invasive electrodes are often used to provide a more exact localization.

Seizures occur during invasive electrode recordings, and care must be used to protect the patient and electrodes during and after the seizures. In many centers, invasive electrodes are used in an intensive care unit. The electrodes may be left in place for days to weeks, depending on the case and how quickly seizures occur.

Subdural electrodes (Fig. 13.1) consist of a series of metal electrodes embedded in plastic and arranged as a strip or a large grid. They cover a large area and record directly from the brain, without interference from the scalp and skull. An operation is required to place these electrodes under the *dura mater*, one of the layers of tissue covering the brain. They do not penetrate the brain. Subdural electrode strips can be inserted through a small hole drilled in the skull, called a "burr hole." In other cases, a section of the skull is removed, the electrodes are put in place, and the skull is replaced or frozen in a sterile location, and the electrodes are covered with the dura mater, the scalp, and a surgical dressing. After the testing is completed, the piece of the skull is replaced. There is a moderate amount of discomfort for several days after electrodes are placed, and medicine is given for pain relief.

The mapping procedures with subdural electrodes involve stimulation of the brain with mild electrical currents to temporarily activate or shut down certain areas. For example, stimulating the left motor cortex controlling the right thumb can cause jerks in this finger, or stimulating language areas in the temporal or frontal lobes can cause a person to suddenly stop speaking. The mapping procedure is almost always painless. If pain occurs, it is momentary and the electrical stimulation can be stopped immediately. The major risks of subdural electrodes are infection (which increases during prolonged use, especially after 6–8 days), bleeding, and brain swelling.

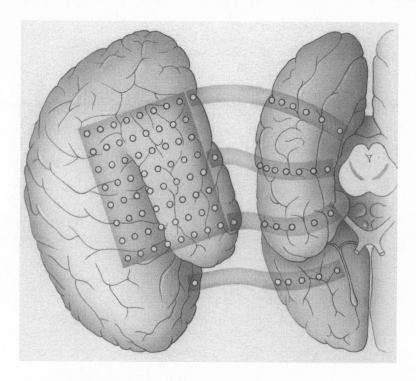

FIGURE 13.1: Subdural electrodes implanted in the brain.

Depth electrodes (Fig. 13.2) are thin, wirelike plastic tubes with metal contact points spread out along their length. Depth electrodes are placed directly into the brain through small burr holes drilled in the skull. The patient is usually awake while the electrodes are being placed, but may be sleeping. The procedure of implanting depth electrodes can be mildly painful since a frame may be used to assist the computerized placement, and placing the frame on the skull can be uncomfortable, but pain medications can be given if needed.

Depth electrodes provide the best recordings of seizures arising in areas deep in the brain, but they also carry some additional risks, especially bleeding within the brain. They are less likely than subdural electrodes to cause infection or brain swelling.

Intracarotid Sodium Amobarbital Test

In the intracarotid sodium amobarbital (Wada) test assesses memory and language functions by putting one hemisphere to sleep

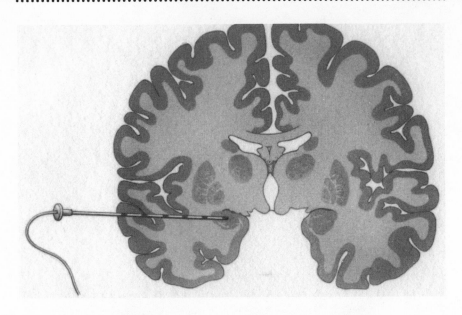

FIGURE 13.2: Depth electrodes implanted in the brain.

with a short-acting anesthetic such as amobarbital and studying what functions are still working in the other hemisphere. The test begins with an angiogram, which examines the flow of a dye through the blood vessels. A thin plastic tube (catheter) is introduced through an artery in the upper thigh. A local anesthetic numbs the area and a needle is inserted into the artery. The tube is threaded through the needle, and the needle is removed. There is some initial mild discomfort, but the rest of the test is painless. The tube is guided up to the carotid artery in the neck. A small amount of contrast dye is injected and x-rays show blood flow in the brain; some warmth or flashing lights may be momentarily experienced.

Next, the anesthetic is given, which puts almost half of brain to sleep for several minutes while language and memory are assessed in the awake cerebral hemisphere. The same procedure is usually repeated on the opposite side after a delay of 30–60 minutes when the patient is fully alert.

The cerebral angiogram test has the possibility of causing a stroke, but the risk is extremely low. The risk is greatest, but still quite low, in older people with atherosclerosis.

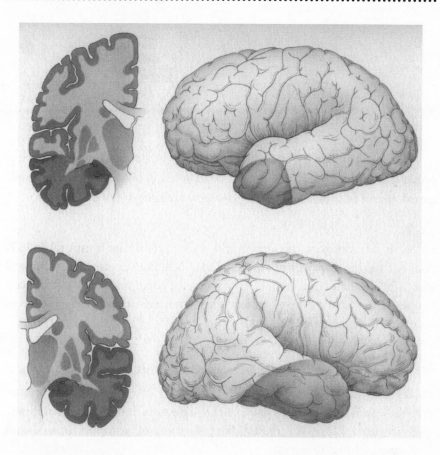

FIGURE 13.3: Brain tissue removed *(shaded areas)* in a standard temporal lobectomy of the left *(top)* or right *(bottom)* hemisphere. (Cross-sectional views, looking from the front, are on the left side of the figure, and side views are on the right.) A smaller amount of tissue is removed from the left hemisphere than from the right hemisphere, because the left temporal lobe contains the area that is vital for language comprehension in most people.

Surgical Procedures

Temporal Lobectomy

Removal of a portion of the temporal lobe (temporal lobectomy) is the most common and most successful type of epilepsy surgery. In most cases, a modest portion is removed, measuring approximately two inches in length (Fig.13.3). The temporal lobes are important in memory and

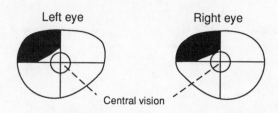

Left eye   Right eye

Central vision

FIGURE 13.4: Superior quandrantanopsia. The patient's central vision is preserved; only the peripheral vision (to the sides) is affected, and most people are unaware of the problem. In most cases, only a portion of this area is affected.

emotion. In addition, the upper and back part of one temporal lobe is vital for language comprehension. This "language-dominant" temporal lobe is on the left in nearly all right-handed people and most left-handed people. Preoperative tests assess the potential impact of surgery on memory or language functions.

The success rate for seizure control varies:

- 60–70% of patients are free of seizures that impair consciousness or cause abnormal movements, but some still experience auras.

- 20–25% of patients have some seizures but are significantly improved (greater than 85% reduction of complex partial and tonic-clonic seizures).

- 10–15% of patients have no worthwhile improvement.

Therefore, more than 85% of patients enjoy a marked improvement in seizure control. Most of them need less medication after surgery. Approximately 25% of those who are seizure-free eventually can discontinue AEDs.

The risk of a major complication such as a stroke, with weakness on the opposite side of the body, is about 1–2% in temporal lobectomy and can vary between surgeons. If the surgery extends to the back part of the temporal lobe, there is also a risk of loss of vision in the upper quarter of space on the side opposite that of the surgery (superior quadrantanopsia) (Fig. 13.4). For example, if the surgeon needs to extend the area of removal toward the back part of the right temporal lobe, a defect in vision in the left upper quarter of space is possible. Luckily, this impairment does not impact daily life and the affected person is usually unaware of it.

If vision was good before surgery, they still can read, drive, and perform tasks requiring extremely precise visual accuracy. In rare cases (fewer than 1 in 200 patients), the visual loss is more severe and includes the half the visual field, on the side opposite the surgery. This impairment (hemianopsia) causes functional problems and interferes with reading and driving.

When surgery is performed on the language-dominant (usually left) side, there is often a mild reduction in memory and retrieval of infrequently used words. After right-sided (nondominant) temporal lobectomy, memory functions are usually stable or may improve slightly. Persons with frequent seizures who achieve complete or nearly complete seizure control and reduced medications after surgery often have better cognitive and mood function. This is especially true for those with problems after individual seizures or clusters of seizures. Overall, there is a significant reduction in depression and anxiety after surgery, although these problems may begin after surgery. Very rarely, psychosis can develop after surgery. The risk of death from temporal lobectomy is approximately 1 in 1000 patients. Note: The risk of psychosis and death from uncontrolled epilepsy is likely greater than from surgery.

If you are taking out a piece of my brain, won't I be a different person?

No. Personality, mood, and overall behavior are hardly ever disrupted or changed by temporal lobectomy. Part of the explanation is that many brain areas perform similar functions. Further, removal or damage to some areas (right frontal or temporal lobes) in previously healthy individuals produces minimal or undetectable effects. For people with uncontrolled seizures, the areas that cause epilepsy and that are removed during surgery are not functioning properly and, in some cases, do not function at all. A pioneer of epilepsy surgery, Wilder Penfield, suggested that the epilepsy tissue is "nociferous," meaning harmful. Therefore, the area from which seizures arise can fail to perform the functions normally served by that area, as well as impair function in other normal brain areas. Removal of nociferous areas may explain improved memory and other cognitive functions in some patients after epilepsy surgery.

Frontal Lobectomy

The frontal lobes comprise approximately one third of the cerebral hemisphere (see Fig. A1.1). This large area is often affected by head trauma, stroke, tumor, and other disorders. Partial seizures often arise in the frontal lobes, the second most common lobe from where resective epilepsy surgery is done.

The back part of the frontal lobes (primary motor cortex) controls movement and cannot be removed without causing severe weakness in muscles on the opposite side. In front of the primary motor cortex is the motor association cortex (Figure A1.1). This area links the primary motor cortex with other brain areas. The motor association cortex can be removed without causing weakness.

It can be challenging to localize a frontal lobe seizure focus. The large size of the frontal lobe and relation of some blood vessels makes it difficult to record electrical activity from all regions. Subdural electrodes sample a greater area of frontal lobe than depth electrodes.

The success rates for frontal lobectomy are not as good as those for temporal lobectomy:

- 40–50% of patients are free of seizures that impair consciousness or cause abnormal movements.

- 20–40% of patients are markedly improved (more than 90% reduction of complex partial and tonic-clonic seizures).

- 10–30% of patients have no improvement or only a mild to moderate improvement.

The risk of major complications, such as a stroke, is about 2%. The risk of behavioral changes is higher than with temporal lobectomy. Behavioral changes associated with frontal lobe impairment are often difficult to measure and define—for example, personality, motivation, ability to plan and to follow up on a multistep process or organize actions over time, and social graces. Some persons with seizures beginning in the frontal lobes may have behavioral problems before the surgery. Behavior can improve after surgery.

Parietal and Occipital Lobectomies

Surgery on the parietal or occipital lobes, located in the back of the brain (see Fig. A1.1), is most often done when a structural abnormality is identified on the CT or MRI scan. The success rate in controlling seizures is higher when a structural abnormality is present. Invasive electrode recordings may reveal or confirm that seizures come from one of these areas.

The successes and risks of parietal and occipital lobectomies are similar to those of frontal lobectomy. The risk of weakness is lower, whereas the risk of impairings touch sensation or vision is greater. On the dominant (usually left) side, the parietal lobe is important in language and skilled motor actions. On the nondominant (usually right) side, the parietal lobe is important for spatial perception and ability to focus attention toward the left side of space. The occipital lobes are essential for vision. The left occipital lobe receives information about vision in the right half of space and vice versa.

Corpus Callosotomy

Corpus callosotomy cuts the large fiber bundle (corpus callosum; see Fig. A1.1B) that connects the two hemispheres of the brain. Unlike lobectomy, corpus callosotomy does not remove brain tissue. The operation usually involves cutting the front two thirds of the callosum to reduce the seizure frequency. Often, a second operation is later performed to cut the remaining back third. Corpus callosotomy is most effective for atonic, tonic-clonic, and tonic seizures. Seizure frequency is reduced by an average of 70–80% after partial callosotomy and 80–90% after complete callosotomy. Partial seizures are often unchanged, but may improve or worsen.

Complications of corpus callosotomy are greater than with lobectomy. Behavioral, language, and other problems may affect function and the quality of life, but serious problems are usually temporary and uncommon. The potential risks of callosotomy must be weighed against its possible benefits, such as a reduction in seizure frequency and AED doses. Behavioral problems after callosotomy are most common when language and motor dominance are controlled by different hemispheres; in left-handed persons, for example, the left side controls language, but the right side controls movement.

Hemispherectomy

The dramatic procedure of hemispherectomy originally involved removing half the brain. Now, it usually involves disconnecting one cerebral hemisphere from the rest of the brain, with removal of only a limited area (Fig. 13.5). It is only considered in patients, usually children, with severe epilepsy in whom seizures arise from only one side of the

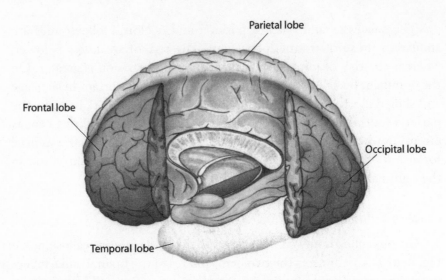

FIGURE 13.5: Side view of the left hemisphere, showing the area of brain removed *(ghost shading)* and the areas of brain disconnected from the opposite hemisphere *(dark shading)* in a hemispherectomy.

brain in which function is very impaired. Before surgery, these patients typically have severe weakness (paralysis) and loss of vision on the opposite side. Therefore, the side of the brain that will be disconnected functions very poorly and the functions of the intact side are compromised by seizures.

If the operation is performed on young children, the opposite hemisphere may make up partly for the loss. They will never have movement or normal sensation in the hand, forearm, foot, and leg on the side opposite the operation. However, controlled movements are possible in the upper arm and thigh, thus permitting the person to walk and use the weak upper limb as a "helper." Physical therapy is often needed after surgery.

Hemispherectomy provides complete or nearly complete seizure control in more than 75% of cases. If the patient has a progressive disorder, such as Rasmussen's syndrome, the prognosis for seizure control is less good.

Multiple Subpial Transections

The multiple subpial transections procedure was pioneered as an alternative to removal of brain tissue. It is used to control partial

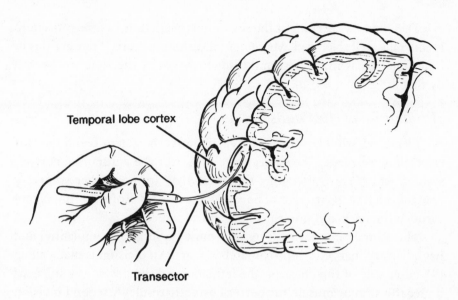

Temporal lobe cortex

Transector

FIGURE 13.6: Multiple subpial transections of the brain.

seizures originating in areas that cannot be safely removed. For example, if the seizure focus involves critical language areas, the removal of this area would devastate language. Similarly, if the seizure focus is in the primary motor area, complete removal would cause permanent weakness.

The operation involves a series of shallow cuts (transections) into the cerebral cortex (Fig. 13.6). The transections are made only as deep as the gray matter, approximately a quarter of an inch. Because of the complex way in which the brain is organized, these cuts are thought to selectively interrupt fibers that connect neighboring parts of the brain. Although the cuts are not quite as selective as we would like (there is microscopic destruction of brain cells), the transections usually do not cause long-lasting problems.

Multiple subpial transections can help reduce or eliminate seizures arising from vital functional cortical areas. Transections can be successfully in Landau-Kleffner syndrome, a disorder in which language problems occur in a child whose language was previously developing normally (see Chapter 3). One concern is that the epileptic activity may recur after a period of 2–20 months. This procedure may achieve long-term reduction in seizure activity, but it is not as effective as removal or disconnection of the seizure focus.

There may be bleeding at the site of the transection, but the procedure is generally well tolerated. Major complications are rare. Transections in functional areas may cause mild impairments in the function served by that area.

Stimulation of the Vagus Nerve

Electrical stimulation of the vagus nerve is a new technique for controlling seizures. The vagus nerve is part of the autonomic nervous system, which controls bodily functions that are not under voluntary control, such as heart rate. The vagus nerve runs from the brainstem through the neck and into the chest and abdomen.

The stimulating device (Fig. 13.7) must be surgically implanted and has a battery that lasts approximately 5 years. An incision is made along the outer side of the chest on the left side, and the device is implanted under the skin or muscle for better cosmetic result. A second incision is made horizontally in the lower neck, along a crease of skin, and the wire from the stimulator is wrapped around the vagus nerve. The procedure takes 45–90 minutes with the patient under general anesthesia, with a hospital stay of one night. However, it may be done under local anesthesia with the patient discharged the same day. The risks of implantation are low. Approximately 1% of implants damage the nerve supplying muscles in the voice box, which can result in permanent hoarseness or a change in voice quality. In addition, when the vagus nerve is stimulated, about one third of patients have some change in their voice quality, which is reversible by reducing the stimulation current or other stimulation features. Even without any change in the level of stimulation, the hoarseness and changes in voice quality often diminish and resolve over weeks or months.

The VNS was approved by the Food and Drug Administration for use in patients with partial epilepsy who are 12 years of age or older. Many centers report success with the device in young children and in patients with primary generalized epilepsy and Lennox-Gastaut syndrome.

The stimulator can be easily activated by holding a magnet near the device. The strength of the current delivered after the magnet is used can be adjusted. For people with warnings (auras) before their seizures, activating the stimulator with the magnet when the warning occurs may help to stop the seizure. However, many patients without auras also show improved seizure control with the vagus nerve stimulator.

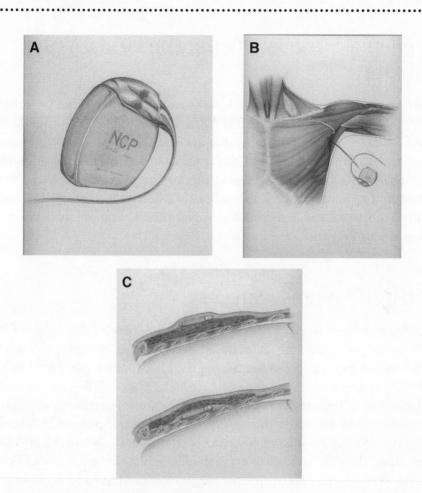

FIGURE 13.7: Vagus nerve stimulator: **(A)** device, **(B)** location of implant, **(C)** under or over pectoralis muscle.

For all patients, the device is programmed to go on for a certain period (for example, 7 or 30 seconds) and then to go off for another period (for example, 14 seconds or 5 minutes). It continuously cycles, intermittently stimulating the vagus nerve throughout the day and night.

Initial controlled studies revealed that after subtracting the "placebo" responses, 20–25% of patients have a 50% or greater reduction in seizure frequency, another one third had their seizures reduced by 20–50%, and the remainder did not have worthwhile improvement. In patients with seizures uncontrolled by AEDs, complete control with the VNS occurs in less than 1%.

Epilepsy Surgery During the First 3 Years of Life

Infants and young children who have seizures that cannot be controlled with medications are surgical candidates. These children usually have MRI evidence of abnormalities that are restricted (or nearly so) to one brain area. In some cases, the abnormality is widespread in one entire hemisphere (e.g., Sturge-Weber syndrome; hemimegalancephaly), and the child's epilepsy is best treated with a hemispherectomy. In most cases, the area is much more limited, and the removal of less tissue can improve or fully control the seizures.

Cost of Epilepsy Surgery

Epilepsy surgery is expensive. Because of the complexities involved in the presurgical planning, it must be performed at an epilepsy center that has an experienced team. Strategies, philosophies, and costs differ among epilepsy centers, depending on the part of the country and the extent of the presurgical assessment. At some centers, for example, patients are monitored with video-EEG for prolonged periods; at others, the monitoring periods are shorter. In addition, if invasive electrodes are used, the cost is much greater than if only a routine video-EEG is done. Overall, the cost of epilepsy surgery varies from $40,000 to more than $100,000. Patients should feel free to ask different centers about their average costs, outcomes, rates of complications, and other factors related to the surgery.

Health insurance covers epilepsy surgery. If the insurance company denies coverage, the patient and the doctor should appeal as surgery is now a standard medical procedure.

III | Epilepsy in Children

14 | Dietary Therapies for Epilepsy

F or centuries, starvation and dehydration were reported to improve seizure control. In addition, substances as diverse as mistletoe, turpentine, and marijuana were claimed to be effective for epilepsy. In 1858, Sir Sieveking wrote, "There is scarcely a substance in the world, capable of passing through the gullet of man, that has not at one time or other enjoyed a reputation of being an anti-epileptic."* In modern times, various vitamins, mineral, amino acids and nutritional supplements are also promoted for epilepsy patients. The ketogenic and Atkins diets are endorsed by medical authorities and can help control seizures in some patients.

The Ketogenic, Modified Atkins, and Low Glycemic Diets

Research in the 1930s showed that a diet consisting mostly of fats dramatically reduced the frequency of seizures in many children. The diet was named the ketogenic diet because it caused a metabolic change called ketosis, whereby the body produces ketone bodies by metabalozing

---

*Sieveking EH: *On Epilepsy and Epileptiform Seizures: Their Causes, Pathology, and Treatment.* J. Churchill, London, 1858, p. 226.

of fat and protein. After the introduction of phenytoin (Dilantin®) in 1938, the ketogenic diet fell out of use, but new studies during the past several decades confirm its value. Several highly publicized dramatic succeses with the ketogenic diet in children whose seizures were not controlled with medications or surgery renewed interest and use. However, the diet is not without side effects—from problems with the child's tolerance for the limited menu to kidney stones, growth retardation, and metabolic disorders. These have led to the use of the modified Atkins and low glycemic (South Beach) diets, which also restrict carbohydrates but allow more protein, thereby increasing tolerability and compliance while also decreasing side effects. Early experience with these less restrictive alternatives to the ketogenic diet suggests that they are effective in some patients.

The Ketogenic Diet
Who is a Candidate?

There are no rules about who is and who is not a candidate for the ketogenic diet. The greatest successes are with children between ages 18 months to 6 years whose seizures cannot be controlled by AEDs, especially with Lennox-Gastaut and Doose syndromes, who have atonic, tonic, and myoclonic seizures. However, all types of seizures can improve. The diet's success depends on the child's previous diet, adaptability, and motivation. After the age of 3–5 years, children have usually been exposed to foods that they are unwilling to part with. Therefore, older children and adolescents need to be highly motivated to stay on the diet. In sensitive patients, "cheating" by eating even small amounts of additional carbohydrates can lead to loss of seizure control. Due to these issues, many parents are hesitant to use the ketogenic diet because their child is a carbohydrate lover or picky eater who barely eats enough. For children with severe epilepsy, however, the potential benefits of a 1- to 3-month trial outweigh the risks. Although this diet can be used successfully in adults, they usually find the modified Atkins or low glycemic diet more tolerable. Infants who are only fed with formula or children who are only fed with a gastrosomy tube can be easily put on the ketogenic diet.

Starting the Diet

The ketogenic diet is most often used in epilepsy centers for children with uncontrolled seizures. The diet should only be started under the co-direction of a physician and a dietician who are familiar with it. Modifications are often needed to make it more effective or tolerable to individual patients. Traditionally (the "Johns Hopkins" approach), the diet is started in the hospital to ensure close supervision and safety. During the first 24–48 hours, there is no food and fluids are limited. This initial period of starvation lowers the child's blood sugar. If the fall in blood sugar is too great, the child may become pale, sweaty, tremulous, irritable, confused, and unresponsive, or may vomit or even have seizures. In such cases, the child requires sugar or other carbohydrate supplementation to prevent more serious side effects. If not monitored closely, fluid restriction may result in dehydration. After starvation, the ketones in the blood and urine rise, and ketogenic food is gradually introduced: one third of the diet on the following day, two thirds the next day, and then the full diet.

Many epilepsy centers initiate the diet outside of the hospital, without the initial starvation or fluid restrictions. This more gradual outpatient regimen has fewer side effects, reduced physical and emotional stress on the patient and family, and reduced costs. Further, the inpatient starvation phase is not tolerated by some patients, who may then forgo the diet that could have been very beneficial. The diet can be monitored with urine ketones measured at home with an indicator strip. Urine ketones show that the diet has achieved its metabolic goal of ketosis; higher ketone levels correlate with improved seizure control in many children.

What is the Diet?

The diet consists primarily of foods high in fat, with most of the remaining calories made up of proteins. With the commonly used 3 or 4:1 ratios of fats to carbohydrates and protein, 70–90% of the foods are fats and 10–30% are carbohydrates and protein. The daily diet often consists of 35–45 calories per pound (75–100 calories/kg) and 0.5–1.0 g of protein per pound (1–2 g/kg) of body weight. Examples of high-fat foods include mayonnaise, butter, and heavy cream. The foods must be carefully measured and weighed. The child is allowed only small portions of cheese, meat, fish, or poultry each day. Fruit is allowed in modest amounts.

Mixed chain triglyceride (MCT), an alternative source of fat, is a clear, light-colored oil that has no flavor. Its use often allows a slight expansion of nonfat foods in the diet. MCT also has laxative properties, beneficial because the ketogenic diet is often constipating. MCT oil should be introduced gradually to avoid stomach cramps.

Because sugar is prohibited in the diet, parents must be vigilant about their children's medications, cough syrups, vitamins, toothpaste, and any other nonfoods or foods that may contain sugar. Small amounts of sugar can reverse the effects of the diet and cause a seizure. All adults who may be with the child in the parents' absence must be informed about the dietary restrictions.

Stopping the Diet

If the diet is well tolerated and effective, the doctor will usually recommend continuing it for 1–3 years. Afterwards, carbohydrates are gradually increased, typically over 2–6 months. Suddenly stopping the diet may cause a temporary increase in seizures.

After the diet is discontinued, some children remain seizure-free without medications. However, seizures may recur, in which case they may be well controlled with medications that were ineffective before the diet. A patient who was seizure-free on a lower ratio of fats to protein and carbohydrates (for example, 2.75:1), but whose seizures recurred when the diet was discontinued, may be helped by continuing the diet at a reduced ratio or trying the modified Atkins or low glycemic diets.

Using AEDs with the Diet

If a child is taking high dosages of several AEDs, tapering of one drug is started around the time the diet is started. If ketosis is maintained and seizure control improves, a further reduction in medications is often possible. Occasionally, all medications can be tapered and stopped. The carbohydrate content of medications, often significant in liquid formulations, must be considered in calculating total carbohydrates.

How successful is the diet?

After 1 year of therapy, approximately one third of patients experience a greater than 50% reduction in seizures (10% are seizure-free), one third have less than a 50% reduction, and one third are unable to tolerate the diet.

What are the possible complications of the diet?

The long-term effects of a high-fat diet, even if it is used for only several years, are unknown. Most experts believe benefits for brain development and intellectual and social functions with improved seizure control and reduced dosages of AEDs outweigh the risks. Many parents worry about the potential effects of large amounts of dietary fat. Although the ketogenic diet raises "bad" lipids (VLDL and

LDL) and lowers "good" lipids (HDL), there is no evidence of increased atherosclerosis in children or adolescents. Weight gain is not usually a problem because caloric intake is carefully supervised.

As previously discussed, the initial starvation period, if used, can cause very low blood sugar levels that require urgent treatment. Other potential problems include a deficiency of the vitamins B, C, and D; calcium; folate; and iron; therefore, these nutrients must be supplemented. The ketogenic diet often slows a child's growth in height and weight, but this is often made up for, at least partially, when the diet is stopped. There is a risk of kidney stones, which can be reduced by adequate fluid intake. Although acetazolamide, topiramate, and zonisamide also predispose to kidney stones, they can still be used with good hydration by patients on the diet. Other complications include constipation and an increased risk of bone fractures.

Where can I get more information?

The Internet provides a rich source of medical and parental wisdom (e.g., epilepsy.com, charliefoundation.org, matthewsfriends.org), but be wary of opinions from one individual or an unknown website. The Internet has everything from recipes and personal observations to supportive chat rooms. There are several informative books: *The Ketogenic Diet: A Treatment for Children and Others with Epilepsy* (by John Freeman et al., 2006), *Keto Kid: Helping Your Child Succeed on the Ketogenic (by Deborah Snider, 2006), and The Ketogenic Diet: A Complete Guide for the Dieter and Practitioner* (by Lyle McDonald and Elzi Volk, 1998). *The Ketogenic Cookbook* (by Dennis and Cynthia Brake, 1997) provides valuable recipes.

The Modified Atkins and Low-Glycemic Diets

Sammy is a 10-year-old boy whose frequent tonic seizures, which began at age 2, finally came under control with the ketogenic diet at age 5 years. Seizures recurred when he was weaned from the diet at age 7 years. He then refused to stay on the ketogenic diet and developed an eating disorder requiring psychological counseling. Seizures recurred off the diet, on higher doses of drugs. At age 8, with his agreement, the modified Atkins diet was started. He remains on it, 2 years later, seizure-free and happy.

The modified Atkins and low-glycemic diets are alternatives to the ketogenic diet. There have been no "head-to-head" comparisons with the ketogenic diet, but available data suggest that they have approximately the same effectiveness with fewer complications and problems. When compared to the ketogenic diet, these diets do not restrict protein intake, total calories, or fluids. They do not require hospitalization, initial fast, or careful calculations and weighing of food. As with the ketogenic diet, both diets produce ketosis; therefore, it can be helpful to monitor urinary ketones with indicator strips. Additionally, these diets are usually much easier for patients to comply with. Finally, the Atkins and low glycemic diets are used by millions of people for weight loss and for diabetes—there is a lot of information about them.

The major advantage of these diets over the ketogenic diet is that they are more like a normal diet, improving tolerability. The unrestricted protein intake is healthier for growing children. Also, although the modified Atkins and low-glycemic diets do not require the high fat content of the ketogenic diet that may accelerate atherosclerosis, the modified Atkins does encourage fat intake. These diets should ideally be used under the supervision of the doctor and with input from a dietician. Weight and height should be monitored, as well as cholesterol and triglyceride levels due to increased fat intake. Possible side effects include weight loss (which may be good!) and, for the modified Atkins diet, elevated cholesterol levels. It is uncertain if kidney stones are increased.

How does the modified Atkins diet differ from the Atkins diet?

The modified form encourages more fat intake and less carbohydrate intake (10–30 g/day) than the original form.

What exactly is the low glycemic index?

The glycemic index is a measure of how quickly a carbohydrate increases the blood sugar level. Carbohydrates with a low glycemic index cause a slower and more gradual increase in blood sugar; those with a high glycemic index a cause more rapid increase in blood sugar. The low glycemic diet encourages carbohydrates with a low glycemic index (<55 on the index; see glycemicindex.com or diabetes.ca/Section_About/glycemic.asp). These carbohydrates also have health benefits by reducing cholesterol and appetite and lowering the risk of diabetes and heart disease. The South Beach diet incorporates low glycemic carbohydrates into the diet. However, in contrast to the Atkins diet, which allows all types of fats, the South Beach diet encourages the healthier, unsaturated fats.

Vitamins, Minerals, and Other Nutritional Supplements

Although many books and websites contain lists of vitamins, amino acids, and other nutritional supplements suggested to control seizures, there is little and often no scientific support for these claims. Unconfirmed reports claim that magnesium, calcium, vitamin E, vitamin B_{12}, melatonin, omega fatty acids, and the amino acids L-taurine, L-tyrosine, or dimethylglycine reduce seizures in some patients. Although patients with deficiencies of some nutrients such as magnesium, calcium, and vitamin B_6 (which rarely causes seizures in newborns) can benefit from supplementation, there is no evidence that they are beneficial for other patients with epilepsy. We really just don't know whether any vitamin, mineral, or other nutritional supplement is generally beneficial or detrimental to seizure control. For example, animal studies suggest that omega fatty acids and melatonin may help control seizures. However, a controlled trial of omega fatty acids in epilepsy patients failed to show any effect. The study does not fully exclude a possible beneficial effect (it may take a longer time or higher dose), but suggests that if such an effect occurs, it is probably small. Some preliminary studies suggest that melatonin may reduce seizure activity in some patients, but controlled studies are lacking. We need more information! One day, researchers may identify a dietary supplement that improves seizure control—we are not there yet.

Nutritional supplements with the amino acids L-taurine and l-tyrosine are recommended for epilepsy patients by many alternative practitioners. Taurine is involved in many cellular functions. It is found naturally in meat, fish, eggs, and dairy products. Taurine is present in many energy drinks and is the ingredient from which Red Bull derives its name. Although taurine may increase inhibitory neurotransmission in some animal studies, the effects of dietary supplementation on the human brain and epilepsy are uncertain. One theoretical concern is if taurine has benefits for epilepsy-that taking it regularly and then missing a dose could cause withdrawal seizures. There are no clearly documented side effects. L-Tyrosine is a critical amino acid in protein synthesis and also forms the building block for several neurotransmitters. There is no evidence that supplementation reduces seizure activity.

There is no nutritional therapy for epilepsy, apart from the ketogenic, modified Atkins and low glycemic diets, for which there is solid evidence for benefits. Western medicine has not studied nutrition as well as it should, and there may well be nutrients that help control seizures. But as of now, there is no proof. However, a multivitamin or specific vitamin or mineral supplement or omega fatty acids in the diet can have other health benefits.

Valproate can deplete the liver's stores of carnitine, a substance that functions like a vitamin to help in fat metabolism. Carnitine supplementation may help prevent the rare cases of liver damage caused by valproate, but this is unproven. Because serious liver damage from valproate is extremely rare, carnitine supplementation should only be considered for individuals at great risk, such as children under age 2 years. Isolated reports suggest that carnitine supplementation can reduce valproate side effects, such as tremor and tiredness, but other controlled studies show no benefit.

Minerals

Minerals are essential nutrients. Very low levels of sodium, calcium, and magnesium can alter the electrical activity of brain cells and cause seizures. Deficiency of these minerals in the diet is rare unless there is severe general malnutrition, but other factors may affect the levels in the body. Low sodium levels may be caused by medications such as diuretics or carbamazepine or oxcarbazepine, by excessive water intake, or by hormonal disorders. Low calcium levels can result from kidney disease or hormonal disorders. Because magnesium levels alter the body's regulation of calcium, low magnesium levels can contribute to or cause low calcium levels. Individuals who chronically abuse alcohol and have poor nutrition often develop low magnesium levels, which can predispose to seizures.

Persons with epilepsy seldom need mineral supplementation for seizure control. Changes in diet or mineral supplements are reasonable for those who have low levels of these minerals.

AEDs that increase liver metabolism (e.g., carbamazepine, phenobarbital, phenytoin, primidone, and valproate) can increase vitamin D metabolism and lead to a deficiency of calcium in the bone. Therefore, combined calcium and vitamin D supplementation may help prevent bone loss. For persons taking these drugs for more than several years, a bone density test can detect this possible complication. If significant reduction of bone density (osteopenia) is found, a consultation with a bone metabolism specialist may be helpful.

Some side effects of valproate may possibly be reduced by mineral supplementation. Inflammation of the pancreas (pancreatitis), which is a rare but serious adverse effect of valproate, may be prevented by selenium supplementation. Selenium at a dose of 100 µg/day was used to prevent valproate-induced pancreatitis in a child who previously had this problem when taking valproate. Selenium (10–20 µg/day) and zinc (30–50 mg/day) also may help to counteract the hair loss that some people experience when taking valproate. These doses are available in many over-the-counter high-potency multivitamins.

15 | Alternative Therapies for Epilepsy

The gaps in knowledge of Western doctors are matched by the range of complementary and alternative therapies (CAM), from spiritual and herbal to nutritional and behavioral therapies. People with epilepsy whose seizures are not fully controlled by AEDs or who experience troublesome side effects often seek help outside the traditional medical boundaries. For others, taking daily medication for years seems intuitively unhealthy and unnatural.

Interest in alternative therapies has grown rapidly in the past few decades. Many patients are interested in therapies such as acupuncture, herbs, carniosacral or chiropractic therapy, and neuroEEG feedback. Which works best? Are there any dangers? Does insurance reimburse for them?

For 99.9% of our species existence, alternative therapies were the only therapies. In many parts of the world, roots, barks, and herbs remain the primary form of medicine. Further, some modern medicines are derived from plants and were once "alternative therapies."

Traditional and alternative approaches diverged as the scientific method became the focus of medicine. Western medicine has failed to adequately study therapies and approaches that do not fit its model of "what should work." In contrast, it has usually excelled in assessing the effectiveness and safety of its treatments. There is an enormous burden of proof required by the FDA for drugs and (less so) for devices to be approved. They must be proven relatively safe and effective. To do this, one must eliminate the powerful effects of bias and placebo.

Bias is the effect of prejudice and expectation. For example, someone who tests a product in which he has a financial interest may consciously or unconsciously slant the interpretation of results. A placebo is a substance whose only effect comes through the power of suggestion. For example, when persons with chest pain caused by heart problems are given a sugar pill (placebo) and told it will make them better, more than 20% report a definite benefit.

When doctors or CAM practitioners prescribe a treatment, they want their therapy to work. To find out whether a treatment is effective and safe, it should be subjected to a rigorous double-blind controlled study in which neither the doctor nor the patient knows which individuals receive the study or other (e.g., placebo) treatment. Unless controlled studies are used, beware! Bias and placebo effects are very powerful. The best doctor's suspicions, hunches, and experiences over several decades of practice can be totally wrong. CAM therapies are rarely subjected to careful scrutiny, especially a double-blind controlled study. Therefore, we unfortunately we do not know whether most of them are helpful, harmful, or simply ineffective.

The book *Complementary and Alternative Therapies in Epilepsy* (Devinsky et al., 2005) reviews an extensive group of CAM approaches in epilepsy. The Internet (www.epilepsy.com, www.epilepsyontario.org) can also provide much information, but many Internet sites should be read with caution, especially when a therapy is promoted by a group that has a financial interest in its use.

The following sections review some common CAM therapies used to treat epilepsy. In addition to those discussed below, homeopathy, osteopathy, craniosacral therapy, traditional Chinese medicine (herbal medicine, acupuncture, moxibustion [burning a processed mugwort herb on the patient's skin]), Ayurveda (ancient Indian medicine), aromatherapy, and hyperbaric oxygen have been used. Again, we lack controlled data as to whether or not of these CAMs improve, worsen, or have no effect on epilepsy.

Drugs are synthetic chemicals and dangerous; alternative therapies are natural and safe.

A common misconception is that if a substance is synthetic, it is unsafe, but if it is natural, it is safe. Hemlock and poisonous mushrooms are deadly, yet very natural plants. In contrast, some synthetic drugs, such as gabapentin, given to millions of people, never caused life-threatening side effects despite even, large overdoses.

Herbal Therapies

Nearly 20% of patients who take prescription drugs also take herbal supplements. Unlike drugs, herbal therapies are classified by the FDA as dietary supplements and are not subject to regulations concerning their preparation, safety, or effectiveness. Herbal therapies are prepared from the flowers, leaves, stems, bark, or roots of plants. Some of these can be taken directly, but others undergo various forms of processing, such as drying of bark. Herbal therapy was used in prehistoric times. Many modern drugs are derived from plants of herbal therapy. Texts from the eighteenth and nineteenth centuries describe many herbal therapies for epilepsy, including mistletoe, foxglove (digitalis), and *Cannabis sativa* (marijuana).

Herbal preparations are often used to treat epilepsy in Asian or African folk medicine practices. The herbal medicines that are alleged, but not proven, to have a beneficial effect on seizures include *Ailanthus altissima* (Tree of Heaven), *Artemisia vulgaris* (mugwort), *Calotropis procera* (calotropis), *Cannabis sativa* (marijuana), *Centella asiatica* (hydrocotyle), *Convallaria majalis* (lily of the valley), *Dictamnus albus* (burning bush), *Paeonia officinalis* (peony), *Scutellaria lateriflora* (scullcap), *Senecio vulgaris* (groundsel), *Taxus baccata* (yew), *Valeriana officinalis* (valerian), and *Viscum album* (mistletoe). Most of these are relatively safe in recommended doses, but side effects include rash, digestive disturbances, and headache. Overdoses can be dangerous.

Some herbal products may cause seizures: ephedra, ginkgo, ginseng, evening primrose, borage, and essential oils such as eucalyptus, fennel, hyssop, pennyroyal, rosemary, sage, savin, tansy, thuja, turpentine, and wormwood. The exact mechanism of how these substances may induce seizures is not known. Ginkgo may reduce the effectiveness of AEDs.

Herbal-AED Interactions

Herbal therapies can interact with AEDs. St John's wort can lower levels of certain AEDs, including phenobarbital and phenytoin. Patients on these AEDs should not use St John's wort. Garlic may increase the levels of some AEDs. Chamomile may intensify or prolong the effects of phenobarbital. Sedating herbs such as kava, valerian, and passionflower can increase sedation produced by phenobarbital, benzodiazepines, and other drugs. Silymarin (milk thistle extract) may increase metabolism and reduce blood levels of valproic acid.

Herbs used as medicinal therapy may cause side effects. In general, most herbal preparations are well tolerated, and if side effects occur, they are mild and improve with continued use. Allergic reactions are possible, as are more serious complications such as liver injury from kava.

Valerian

Valerian is a flowering plant used as a sedative to treat insomnia and anxiety. Although recommended by some as a therapy for epilepsy, no solid evidence supports this use. Although it appears safe, consuming large doses for sustained periods may lead to tolerance, and withdrawal symptoms may occur when it is stopped.

Kava

Kava is a plant used in medical as well as social and religious practices in Pacific cultures for thousands of years. Currently, it is recommended for anxiety and stress, although it is also being studied as a treatment for cancer. Although some evidence suggests that kava can alter ion channels and GABA activity, similar to AEDs, there is no evidence that kava improves seizure control. Recent reports of liver damage from kava have limited its use.

St John's Wort

St John's wort (*Hypericum*) is a flowering plant that is mainly used to treat depression and, to a lesser extent, anxiety. Controlled studies show that St John's wort does improve symptoms of mild, but not moderate to severe, depression. Like many antidepressants (such as Zoloft and Lexapro), St John's wort appears to increase brain serotonin levels. Side effects tend to be mild and include stomach discomfort, dizziness, tiredness, headache, dry mouth, and sexual dysfunction.

Ginkgo Biloba

Leaves from ginkgo trees contain a variety of compounds that help increase blood flow to body tissues, serve as antioxidants, and reduce blood clotting. Ginkgo is often recommended to improve memory. There is some data that it can produce mild improvement in memory in patients with Alzhehimer's disease, but that data is not conclusive. It is usually well tolerated, but headache, nausea, vomiting, and diarrhea can occur. An increased risk of bleeding is possible. There are isolated cases of seizures with ginkgo use, but these are rare and not confirmed. There is no evidence that ginkgo improves seizure control.

Ephedra

Ephedra is a chemical derived from the *Ephedra sinca* plant. It is a brain and cardiovascular stimulant that was used to promote weight loss (with some short-term but no long-term benefits), but is now illegal in the United States due to serious side effects, including seizures and death.

Relaxation Therapy and Biofeedback

> Susan had a history of chronic epilepsy and was not controlled after trials of eight different AEDs. During her evaluation for epilepsy surgery, her husband of 15 years filed for divorce and moved out of their home. Two weeks later, her complex partial seizures, documented on video-EEG recordings, were reduced from four per week to less than one per 6 months. The end of her stressful marriage did more for her seizure control than any AED.

Many adults with epilepsy report that stress can provoke a seizure. Because stress can alter brain chemistry and electrical activity, stress may worsen epilepsy in susceptible people. It can also cause sleep deprivation and rapid breathing, which makes seizures more likely in some people.

Relaxation therapy involves a variety of strategies to reduce stress and foster relaxation. Breathing exercises, hypnosis, and other techniques can be employed. Biofeedback involves learning to control bodily functions that are usually not under voluntary control. One can learn to control these functions by providing information about them to conscious awareness. For example, the heart rate can be modified by listening to a beep every time one's heart beats and concentrating on lowering or raising the heart rate. Similarly, biofeedback can lower the tension in the facial muscles or slow the breathing rate.

Both relaxation therapy and biofeedback can help to improve seizure control in some persons by reducing stress and controlling hyperventilation, but they rarely make someone seizure-free. Tai chi, yoga, and therapeutic massage can also help relieve stress. We need systematic study of these techniques in epilepsy to better define their role.

Neurofeedback (neuro-EEG feedback, neurotherapy) uses operant conditioning of the brain's electrical activity (EEG) to try and reduce seizure activity. Unlike many CAM therapies, there is good basic science to support this technique. First, a quantitative EEG is obtained to identify abnormal brain rhythms. These rhythms are then targeted with conditioning exercises to make them more normal and thereby hopefully reduce seizure activity. The sessions typically last about 1 hour, occur one to three times per week, and last for 3-12 months. Neurofeedback is a promising technique that has become more popular, although we do not have controlled data to support its use in epilepsy.

Acupuncture

Acupuncture is used in China and by some practitioners in the West to treat seizures. Acupuncture can alter nervous system activity and can substitute for anesthetic drugs in some surgical procedures. Using acupuncture instead of anesthetic drugs. The ways in which acupuncture works are poorly understood, and there are no well-designed studies that show that acupuncture is effective for epilepsy.

Chiropractic Therapy

Some chiropractic teachings suggest that specific nutrients or forms of spinal manipulation can improve seizure control. There is no evidence to support these claims.

Self-Control of Seizures

Many epilepsy patients have warnings of their seizures and have learned techniques to "fight off a seizure." The warnings may be premonitory symptoms that occur 20 minutes to several days before a seizure. Such symptoms may include irritability, depression, fatigue, "not feeling right," or a headache. Patients with well-defined premonitory symptoms may prevent a seizure from occurring by getting more sleep or taking additional medication (a "rescue" medicine such as lorazepam) under a doctor's supervision.

Some patients have simple partial or myoclonic seizures that occur seconds to minutes before a seizure and report being able to "block" the seizure from progressing. How an individual stops a seizure from progressing is often hard to describe, but it is a real phenomenon. Some patients need to "focus on a difficult problem," "get up and walk," "relax," or keep repeating to themselves "no, no, no." Some patients who experience a tingling sensation or jerking movement in an arm or leg can prevent a tonic-clonic seizure by vigorously rubbing or scratching the arm or leg. Similarly, some patients with seizures beginning with a smell (olfactory aura) can stop their seizure from progressing by smelling an unrelated strong odor. More examples of self-control of seizures appear in the book *Epilepsy: A New Approach,* by Adrienne Richard and Joel Reiter.

16 | Epilepsy in Infancy

A new child is a bundle of joy, anticipation, and expectations. Any illness that the child may have, especially epilepsy, can devastate the parents and family. Seizures in a newborn usually subside quickly but may recur in later childhood. The greatest challenge is fear of the unknown. If the cause of the seizures is understood, the doctor can better predict the baby's development than if the cause is unknown. Even if no cause can be found, however, and all diagnostic tests are normal, there is an excellent chance that the baby will develop normally.

Seizures Newborns

Jane was 2 days old, on a respirator in the intensive care unit. I was so afraid she wouldn't live or, if she did, that there would be permanent brain damage. Then they told me that she was having seizures and needed phenobarbital. It was all very frightening, but Janey is now 2 years old, has been off phenobarbital since 6 months, and has not had any seizures since leaving the hospital at 2 weeks of age.

Seizures in newborns (the first month of life) may appear as fragments of seizures in older children. The infant's brain is still developing and cannot make the coordinated responses of a tonic-clonic seizure. The baby may have jerking or stiffening of a leg or an arm that alternates from side to side, or the whole upper body may suddenly jerk forward, or both legs may jerk up toward the belly with the knees bent. The baby's facial expression, breathing, and heart rate may change. Impairment of responsiveness, which is critical in defining many types of seizures in children and adults, is difficult to assess in newborns. Parents may suspect that responsiveness is impaired when their voices cannot attract the newborn's attention or when the luster in their baby's eyes is replaced by a glaze.

Even experts have difficulty in recognizing seizures in newborns. Neurologists are often told not to watch their own babies and young children too closely, especially when they sleep, because even they may mistake normal gestures for seizures. Normal babies have many sudden, brief jerks, grimaces, stares, and mouth movements that might suggest a seizure. A seizure is more likely if the behavioral changes are repetitive and identical in their features and duration, if the episodes are not brought on by changes in posture or activity, and if the behaviors are not typical of children of the same age. Videotape the suspected behavior for the doctor to review. The EEG is very helpful in defining seizures, but is more difficult to interpret in newborns.

The Moro reflex in babies is a normal response that can be easily mistaken for a seizure. When a baby is startled, such as by momentary removal of support of its head, a loud noise, or a bright light, its spine will stiffen, its arms and legs will extend outward from the body, and its fingers will fan out. The Moro reflex is present in its full form until age 3 months and in an incomplete form until age 5 months. Another normal infant behavior is jitters or shivering movements or tremors.

Newborns with a rare genetic disorder, benign familial neonatal convulsions, have frequent brief seizures in the first few days of life. The disorder usually is inherited by an autosomal dominant gene (that is, one parent also had the disorder), but it may also result from a spontaneous mutation in the child's DNA. The seizures usually stop by 9 months of age.

Seizures in Infants

> I just knew something was not right. My other children had sudden jerks when they were startled and sometimes when they slept, but Jessie's jerks happened while he was awake, just watching a mobile. The pediatrician said not to worry, but when his whole body stiffened, the doctor ordered an EEG, and it showed epilepsy waves.

Seizures in infants (babies from age 1 to 12 months) are similar to those that occur in newborns. Because older infants are able to focus their attention briefly, parents and doctors can better identify impaired consciousness during seizures. Some seizures are episodes of staring from which the infant cannot be distracted. Normal children daydream, but it may be difficult to distract the healthiest of babies at times; seizures cannot be diagnosed simply because the child stares. During some seizures, the infant may suddenly stiffen or jerk or lose muscle tone and become limp. With other seizures, the baby may make repetitive movements that appear semi-purposeful. At times, the seizure may be more violent, and the baby may fall, or its entire body may stiffen and jerk. Because breathing may be briefly interrupted or irregular, the face may become pale or blue, but the seizure is almost never life-threatening.

Nearly all seizures in infants last less than 5 minutes. If seizures last more than 5 minutes or occur in a series, the baby should be taken to an emergency room unless a specific therapy and plan were previously discussed with the doctor.

An uncommon disorder called *infantile spasms* (West's syndrome) usually develops during infancy and lasts an average of 5–6 months with treatment (see Chapter 3). Many of these children will later have developmental delays and other seizures.

Febrile seizures are tonic-clonic seizures that may occur in infants and young children when they have a high fever (see Chapter 3).

Diagnosis of Newborn and Infant Seizures

Doctors try to identify the cause of seizures in newborns and infants. Commonly recognized causes of seizures before the age of 1 year include fever, birth injury and trauma, birth defects resulting from abnormal brain development in the womb, genetic and metabolic disorders, encephalitis (viral infection of the brain), and bacterial meningitis (infection of the brain's membranes). Depending on the baby's medical history and examination, the doctor may order a variety of tests or procedures to look for:

- Structural abnormalities in the brain, using an ultra-sound, CT scan, or MRI

- Abnormal electrical activity in the brain, using an EEG

- Metabolic problems, testing blood, urine, and possibly spinal fluid

- Genetic disorders, using chromosomal studies

- Evidence of infection or metabolic disorders, using a spinal tap (lumbar puncture)

The lumbar puncture provides a sample of spinal fluid. It is safe and not very painful. The baby's worst crying usually comes when the doctor cleans the skin with a cool antiseptic solution. An anesthetic cream can be used on the skin.

In many cases no cause can be found. Brain injuries causing seizures may be impossible to pinpoint, especially injuries with only microscopic damage.

Rarely, seizures in newborns and infants result from a vitamin B_6 (pyridoxine) deficiency. It is important to recognize the deficiency because it is a very treatable. The diagnosis can be established by recording the EEG while injecting vitamin B_6. An improvement in the EEG patterns indicates a vitamin B_6 deficiency.

Treatment of Seizures in Newborns and Infants

The treatment of seizures in newborns and infants is determined by the type of seizure and its cause. In some cases no therapy is needed because the seizure is an isolated event, such as a febrile seizure. In other cases replacement of a missing nutrient can stop further seizures, as in low blood sugar levels or a calcium or vitamin B_6 deficiency.

Usually, babies with epilepsy must be treated with AEDs. As with any other age group, doctors try to balance the benefits of seizure control against the side effects. They sometimes prefer to keep the dosage low and let the baby have a brief seizure once a week, rather than use a high dosage that provides seizure-freedom as well as sedation.

If a baby with epilepsy is developmentally delayed, what is causing the delay—the seizures, the epilepsy waves found on the EEG, the medicines, or the underlying problem? This question is difficult to answer, and multiple factors may be responsible. To further complicate our understanding, when one factor changes, it can change the others. For example, lowering the dosage and the number of AEDs may reduce side effects but increase the epilepsy waves and seizures. MRI may show a structural problem that is the major cause of the developmental delay, but such babies also may be extra sensitive to the effects of seizures and medications. Despite the challenges, these questions should be addressed.

Pediatricians and family physicians are often the first to diagnose seizures, but these infants should be evaluated by a pediatric neurologist or epilepsy specialist.

17 | Epilepsy in Childhood

Causes of Epilepsy in Childhood

Seizures and epilepsy in children have many causes. Common causes include fever, genetic factors, infections of the brain and its coverings, brain damage due to lack of oxygen or trauma, hydrocephalus (excess water in brain cavities), disorders of brain development, and metabolic disorders. Less common causes of childhood epilepsy include brain tumors or cysts and degenerative disorders (progressive conditions, often associated with loss of brain cells). There is an important difference between something that causes seizures, such as a high fever in a young child, and something that causes epilepsy, such as a brain injury or infection.

Extensive and careful studies have not found evidence that immunizations cause epilepsy. However, a seizure may occur within days of an immunization, especially if it is followed by a fever. Such cases are probably innocent febrile seizures. When the child receives subsequent immunizations, the parents should ask the doctor about using acetaminophen (Tylenol) or ibuprofen (Advil, Motrin) before a fever develops. Children who have a single seizure following an immunization can usually receive further immunizations.

Many childhood seizures are benign: they stop without treatment and the child's development and intellect are normal. Other seizures are serious and often are associated with developmental delay or mental retardation and persistent seizures. The outlook for seizures only partially depends on their cause. For example, two children may be infected with the same bacteria and both have meningitis, an infection of the membranes covering the brain and spinal cord. One child develops severe epilepsy, but the other child never has a seizure. How can the different outcomes be explained? The infection in one child may have been more severe, involving sensitive areas of the brain. Or the bacteria could have infected a vein in one child and caused a small stroke, which then caused the epilepsy. Or one child may have a genetic tendency to have seizures aggravated by the infection.

All people are capable of having a seizure. It remains uncertain why some children have seizures after incidents such as moderate head trauma while most others do not. "Seizure threshold" refers to the conditions necessary to produce a seizure. In animals, the seizure threshold can be precisely defined with chemicals or electrical stimulation. In humans, "seizure threshold" is used more abstractly. A person with a low seizure threshold has a lower tendency to have seizures; a higher threshold indicates a greater resistance against seizures. Genetic, hormonal, sleep, and other factors can influence an individual's seizure threshold.

Making the Diagnosis of Epilepsy in Children

My son's teacher noticed Bobby zoning out during class and that his academic performance was declining. Initially, she thought he was just daydreaming, but once he stopped speaking, blinked his eyes, and didn't respond when she called his name. I had seen him do it when he was tired. The pediatric neurologist did an EEG and when he was blowing to make the pinwheel spin, he had an absence seizure. On a prolonged EEG, it turned out Bobby was having as many as 20 a day! The good news is that he may grow out of it, but until then he'll need to take medication.

Epilepsy is diagnosed when a child has two or more seizures that are not provoked by reversible cause such as very low blood sugar. A detailed history of a child's episodes is the most helpful tool for making the diagnosis of epilepsy (see Chapter 9). The doctor will want to know how the episode began and what happened. Did the spell begin suddenly, during exposure to flickering lights, or after an argument? Was consciousness impaired? Were there jerking movements, automatic chewing or hand movements, eye deviation or blinking, or loss of bladder control? Afterward, did the child go to sleep? Or act confused? How long did the episode last? (It is best to time an episode with a watch.) Record a video of an episode for the doctor to view. All of this information will help to determine if the episode was a seizure and, if so, what type.

Obtaining an accurate description of symptoms that a child experiences during a seizure is an art. Note features like facial expression of fear, or comments that "my tummy hurts" just before a seizure; the child is likely experiencing a partial seizure with an emotion of fear and abdominal discomfort. For some symptoms, only the child can tell you what they feel. Many children fail to report symptoms because of shyness, embarrassment, inability to put experiences such as déjà vu into words, inability to recall the event, etc. If simply asked what he or she experiences, such a child may just shrug. When given a choice of possible symptoms, however, the child will often say that one or more occurred before the seizure, even if they did not! The challenge is to separate true from imaginary symptoms. Therefore, all children who can talk about their symptoms should first be asked in a nonthreatening way if they feel anything before or during the spell, or if they ever have sudden, strange feelings separate from it, which could possibly be a simple partial seizure. If they answer no, inquiries should be made about specific symptoms.

Conditions Confused with Childhood Seizures

Not every event that involves jerking, staring, or impairment of consciousness is a seizure. Many behaviors mimic seizures, and it may take time and testing to sort out which are seizures.

Daydreaming

We all daydream, and children daydream more than adults. Daydreaming in children can be easily confused with absence or complex partial seizures, in which staring is a prominent feature. However, lip smacking, eye blinking, grimacing, or stiffening of muscle groups is common during seizures but not during daydreaming. Daydreaming can be stopped by calling the child's name, producing a startling noise, tickling, saying "Look at the kitty" or "fire truck," or shutting off the TV. Absence and complex partial seizures seldom stop by such means, although the child may be partially responsive. Absence seizures usually last less than 10 seconds, and complex partial seizures, 30 seconds to 3 minutes. Daydreaming tends to occur when the child is tired or bored or is involved in monotonous activity, such as riding in a car; seizures can occur at any time. Seizures begin abruptly and often unnaturally (for example, in the middle of a sentence or playing with a toy), while daydreaming often is a continuation of a natural pause in activity such as reading.

"Blue" Breath-Holding Spells

In a classic "blue" breath-holding spell, a young child cries intensely for a long time (usually after some minor upset such as a bump on the head, being scolded, or when a toy is taken away), holds her breath, and then loses consciousness and becomes limp. The child often turns bluish and may sweat profusely. The typical attack lasts 30–60 seconds. With more prolonged spells, the entire body may become rigid and jerk, as the lack of oxygen to the brain actually triggers a seizure. Although it looks like an epileptic seizure, the child does not have epilepsy. The typical sequence of a physical or emotional upset, followed by crying and breath-holding is key in diagnosis. Breath-holding spells do not cause brain injury.

Breath-holding spells usually begin between 6 and 18 months of age and stop before the child is 6 years old. About 25% of the patients have a family history of breath-holding spells. The outlook is excellent and treatment is rarely needed. Distracting the child during the intense crying can prevent the spell. Parents of children who are prone to prolonged vigorous crying tantrums should try to ignore the behavior, withholding the attention and concern that reinforces it. In some cases, a psychologist may help in modifying the child's behavior.

Pallid Infantile Syncope

Syncope (SIN-ko-pee) means fainting. Pallid infantile syncope may be confused with atonic, tonic, or tonic-clonic seizures. The child suddenly becomes pale (pallid) and then faints. Often family members have had similar spells in early childhood, sometimes called "pallid breath-holding spells." In contrast to breath-holding spells, episodes are not always preceded by intense crying. If the spells are prolonged, the entire body may become rigid and jerk as the lack of oxygen to the brain triggers a seizure. This disorder usually begins between 12 and 18 months of age and ends before age 6. The prognosis is excellent and treatment is rarely needed.

Other Forms of Fainting

Fainting is common in children. In many cases, other family members have a history of fainting. Painful or stressful situations such as having blood drawn or watching an upsetting scene can cause a child to faint. Children also may faint from the dehydration caused by inadequate fluid intake or excessive fluid loss from sweating or diarrhea. In other cases, heart disorders causing irregularities of the heartbeat are responsible. Lightheadedness, dizziness, or impaired vision often precedes the faint. Recovery is rapid; confusion or tiredness usually resolves within minutes. Frequent episodes of fainting should be thoroughly investigated by a doctor.

Movement Disorders

Many movement disorders can be confused with tonic or motor seizures. Children with these disorders assume abnormal postures (parts of their bodies are in an unusual position, such as the fingers curled up as if in a cramp, or the foot turned inward) or make sudden, unusual movements (such as eye blinking or jerks of a body part), and the attacks may begin suddenly, thus mimicking seizures. Most of these movement disorders occur spontaneously, but others are triggered by specific events such as eating (Sandifer's syndrome).

Tics are involuntary, repetitive, intermittent, brief movements; they are not seizures. Although tics are purposeless, they may resemble purposeful movements. The most common tics in children are eye blinks, facial grimaces, shoulder shrugs, and head movements. The most severe form is Tourette's syndrome, which is also associated with vocal tics ranging from grunts and throat-clearing sounds to involuntary cursing.

Sleep jerks (benign nocturnal myoclonus) are brief, involuntary muscular contractions that occur as a person falls asleep. In some cases, they may awaken someone who is drifting off to sleep. Sleep jerks are common in healthy children and adults but may be confused with myoclonic seizures.

Taking Medications

Young children often hate taking medications but can usually be coaxed. It may be necessary to crush the pills and put the powder in the child's favorite foods, add liquid medication to something pleasant tasting such as chocolate syrup, or give the child a small reward if he or she takes the liquid or pills. Even small children can understand the importance of taking their pills: it will help keep them well. Older children can understand that they are taking medicine to prevent seizures. Parents may want to use themselves as an example. They might take a vitamin so the children can copy their behavior. *Caution: Keep all medications out of the reach of young children.*

Many children and adolescents feel that they are unable to swallow medication in a tablet or capsule form. Although chewable, sprinkle, and liquid formulations are often available, a child can practice taking tablets or capsules by learning to swallow a mini or whole M&M or Tic-Tac candy with a chewed-up cookie. Alternatively, the pill can be placed on the back of the tongue and taken with water or juice from a glass rather than bending over a drinking fountain. Medication can also be mixed with a food or taken just when a mouthful of food has been chewed ("to a pulp") and then swallowed.

When a child with epilepsy is away from home, whether visiting the grandparents for the weekend or going to summer camp, the medication schedule should be maintained. The child, parent, or both can organize a medication box filled with the necessary number of doses and the times for taking them. Alternatively, a company called Medicine-on-Time (medicine-on-time.com; 800-722-8824) will bubble-pack individual medication doses and label them by date and time.

Video Games and Epilepsy

Media reports have heightened public awareness that playing video games can rarely trigger seizures, but video games do not cause epilepsy. Playing video games is a common and prolonged activity for many kids. Because epilepsy is a common disorder, some seizures while playing video games are coincidental.

Children who are photosensitive, in whom flashing lights or flickering images can trigger seizures or epilepsy waves on the EEG, may have seizures caused by playing video games. Photosensitivity occurs in only 3% of people with epilepsy, so almost all children who have epilepsy should be able to play video games without ill effects. Don't restrict a child from playing video games simply because he or she has epilepsy.

Parents who are unsure whether a child who has epilepsy is photosensitive should check with the doctor. Photosensitive children may be able to play some games quite safely but have problems with others. Medication can often prevent seizures caused by photosensitivity.

For concerned parents, observe the child during the game, looking for lapses in awareness or for rapid blinking or twitching of the mouth or face, jerking movements of other parts of the body. Although one or more of these signs does not necessarily mean that a child has epilepsy or is photosensitive, tell your doctor. Also, consult your doctor if a child has strange or uncomfortable sensations caused by light shimmering on water, sunlight flickering through the trees, or flashing strobe lights, or any usual reaction to sudden or strong light.

The following suggestions, adapted from ways of reducing the risk of seizures in photosensitive children while they watch television or use computers, may help with regard to video games:

- Play in a well-lighted room to reduce the contrast between the lighted screen and the surrounding area. Reducing the brightness of the screen may also be helpful.

- Keep as far back from the screen as possible.

- Use smaller screens in which it is more difficult to see the horizontal scan lines.

- Avoid playing for long periods.

≈ Take regular breaks, and look away from the screen every once in a while.

≈ Cover one eye while playing, alternating between the right eye and the left eye (only consider this for children with known photosensitivity).

≈ Stop the game if strange or unusual feelings develop.

18 | Epilepsy in Adolescence

The passage from childhood to adulthood is surrounded by issues of rebellion, indepen dence, heightened self-consciousness, experimentation, dating, driving, and concerns for the future. Adolescents and their parents share the highs and lows of this often stormy period, and communication between them is essential to temper its turbulence. This is a challenge for both parents and adolescents as intense emotions and feelings create conflicts; parents are heroes and villains, best friends and "police officers," and sources of great affection and frustration.

The adolescents' tidal waves of emotions can consume them and those around them. Emotions are infectious. Parents must maintain their perspective and remain sensitive to their child's insecurities, peer pressures, and need for support. The parents must communicate with their children about drugs, smoking, drinking, and sexually transmitted diseases. The key to communication is allowing children to be comfortable opening up. Becoming judgmental too quickly can damage trust and openness. Parents need to educate their children and share their feelings, but in a positive manner. If adolescents engage in dangerous or irresponsible activities, parents may need to "read them the riot act," but they should try to pause first before reacting in their own emotional storm. Adolescents often know when they have done something wrong and are embarrassed and frustrated by their actions.

Adolescence does not need any complicating factors, but epilepsy is just that. In a time of life marked by continuous adjustments to dramatic physical, mental, social, and academic changes, epilepsy can upset the tenuous balance. Epilepsy, even if it is well controlled, can torment adolescents, arousing fears of or actual isolation and stigma fed by their heightened self-consciousness and exaggerated concerns over physical and social image. Restrictions on activities can accentuate differences from others. For children entering adolescence with good self-esteem and a sense of independence, the impact of epilepsy can be minimal. But epilepsy can aggravate or create problems of low self-esteem, dependency, or behavioral difficulties.

Puberty

Puberty marks the sexual transition from childhood to adolescence. The sex hormones initiate physical and mental changes. The age at which puberty begins varies considerably; children who have early or late changes are often concerned, and sometimes teased, about the differences in their bodies and their schoolmates.

The sex hormones affect the body *and* the brain, altering electrical and chemical activity, personality, mood, and, in some cases, seizure activity. Hormone release is both continuous and episodic; there are periods when large amounts are released over short periods, causing relatively rapid changes in mood and physical features.

Seizures may begin or stop or change around puberty. This relationship may be coincidental, but hormonal changes are likely involved in some cases. Hormones such as estrogen may increase the likelihood of seizures, and many women report that seizures most often occur around their menstrual and ovulatory periods (see Chapter 7). Rapid changes in growth during puberty can alter AED blood levels. If seizure control worsens, the possibility of a decrease in AED levels should be considered.

Taking Medications

> I know Steve doesn't take his medication regularly. I try to remind him every morning and every night. It's more than forgetting. By not taking his medications, he is saying, "I don't really have epilepsy." I hope he realizes that he won't be able to drive if he still has complex partial seizures.

Maturity should make adolescents more aware of the benefits of taking AEDs. For some, however, rebellion or denial dominates, making them less compliant. Adolescents can usually understand the consequences of taking or not taking their medications. Education about AEDs can come from both the parents and the doctor, but the adolescent should be enlisted as an active partner in his or her treatment. Teenagers with epilepsy should take greater responsibility for their care. It may help for the adolescent and doctor to be alone for part of each visit, fostering independence, a sense of self-control, and trust with the doctor and the parents.

With older children and adolescents, the easiest and the best assessment of compliance is simply to ask them straight out: "Are you taking your medication?" Measuring the AED blood levels at intervals can tell the doctor and the parents if the medications were taken as prescribed and can reinforce compliance. However, problems with drug absorption or metabolism, or a period of rapid growth in height and weight, can cause lower levels.

Driving

Driving a motor vehicle is an act of independence. The "driving birthday" is very special. Many people with epilepsy can drive, but there are safety concerns and legal issues that limit driving for many people with epilepsy (see Chapter 25). In most states, a person with epilepsy must submit a letter or form from the doctor about his or her seizure disorder. Many states ask the doctor about their recommendation, which is influenced by compliance with medications: remind adolescents that a favorable report depends on their taking the medications as prescribed.

As the age for driving approaches, review the adolescent's medical care. If no seizures have occurred for several years, it may be wise to attempt to lower and eventually stop medications at least 6 months or a year before the driving age. If the adolescent's seizures are poorly controlled, however, approaching the legal age for driving may prompt referral to an epilepsy center for reevaluation and possible changes in therapy. Adolescents with uncontrolled seizures that affect consciousness or motor control cannot obtain a driver's license.

Dating

Dating does not come naturally to most people. Adolescents are often uncomfortable or uneasy when they start to date, and epilepsy is often a complicating factor. Although epilepsy should be discussed with anyone who is being dated regularly, it is reasonable to wait until the relationship feels comfortable. The person should not be tested. For example, don't make up "people you know with epilepsy" to see how the other person reacts. If the discussion is open and honest, friends will be more willing to ask questions and share their feelings. If the adolescent's seizures are not well controlled, however, discuss epilepsy sooner rather than later, and preferably in person.

Every person who has asked someone for a date has known the fear of possible rejection. Someone with epilepsy has the added fear that he or she will be rejected because of the epilepsy. This fear is not completely unfounded. Some people who hear the word epilepsy become frightened, a fear based on lack of knowledge. But they can be educated. Their understanding of epilepsy and feelings about it will reflect those of the person who lives with it: if the person with epilepsy is comfortable in discussing it, those around them will usually be supportive and comfortable.

Rejection is part of the dating game. No one is spared. People are rejected for many reasons. Although epilepsy is one of many possible reasons that someone may reject someone else, often it is not *the* reason.

Sexual Activity

As one grows closer in a relationship, there is a natural tendency to have intimate contact. There is no reason to fear having a seizure during kissing or other intimate contact any more than at other times, but intimate contact does not protect someone from a seizure. The more frequent the seizures, the more likely a seizure may occur during intimate contact, so the partner should know what to do if a seizure occurs.

Although the vast majority of people with epilepsy are able to enjoy sexual feelings and activities, some have less interest in sexual activity than their peers. The libido, or interest in sexual activity, may be affected by some AEDs, especially those that activate liver enzymes (for example, carbamazepine, phenytoin, phenobarbital), or possibly by the epilepsy itself. The person with epilepsy is often not aware of a problem. Instead, it may be noticed by a parent or significant other. If it does become an issue, it may be helpful to discuss it with a doctor since changing medications or reducing the dosage may be helpful.

Use of Alcohol and Illegal Drugs

When adolescents use alcohol or illegal drugs, trouble is not far behind. Their immaturity, impulsivity, and willingness to take chances often put adolescents who use alcohol or other drugs in particularly dangerous situation, such as driving or sex. Few adolescents fully understand the potential dangers of drugs. Alcohol is the leading cause of motor vehicle accidents in the United States, and teenage drivers in fatal accidents are more likely to have used alcohol than other age groups. Cocaine can cause strokes, heart attacks, seizures, or death.

The rules concerning alcohol use and epilepsy apply to both adolescents and adults, but greater caution applies to the younger group. One or two alcoholic beverages usually cause no meaningful changes in AED levels or in seizure control. The problem is that one or two drinks become three or four, intoxication clouds judgment, and serious problems can follow. Teenagers often will sleep off a hangover, and those with epilepsy may fail to take their bedtime and morning medications. Adolescents with epilepsy should know that alcohol use can worsen seizure control. In addition, the combination of AEDs and alcohol can be very sedating. Teenagers with epilepsy should not drink alcohol, smoke marijuana, or take other drugs.

Cocaine can cause seizures in someone who has never had one before and worsen seizure control in someone with epilepsy. Seizures associated with cocaine use are much more dangerous than seizures that occur from other causes or spontaneously, and they can be fatal. Seizures can be caused or made worse by the use of stimulants (amphetamines), heroin or other opiates, LSD ("acid"), PCP ("angel dust"), "ecstasy," or the withdrawal of sedative-anxiety drugs such as benzodiazepines and barbiturates. These drugs are illegal and very dangerous for adolescents with epilepsy.

Thinking About a Career

Although most adolescents don't choose their future career in high school, some thought to their future is often helpful. Certain classes in high school or college can advance knowledge and skills related to an area of interest. Guidance counselors and vocational counselors often are available in high school to discuss career plans.

Persons with well-controlled or infrequent seizures should have few or no limitations on possible careers, but those with uncontrolled seizures may face some limitations. Adolescents with epilepsy and developmental disabilities such as mental retardation, cerebral palsy, or blindness now have greater work opportunities (see Chapter 28). Realistic but progressive and positive expectations are critical.

Part-Time Employment

Part-time work can be rewarding for adolescents who have epilepsy. In addition to their paycheck, work can provide discipline, skills, education, and a sense of accomplishment and success. A part-time job is often an important step toward independence. The job should be balanced in the child's academic and social life; sleep deprivation or the stress of overwork can increase seizure frequency.

19 | Outgrowing Epilepsy

S lightly more than half of the children who have epilepsy
outgrow it. This simple and positive fact raises important
questions: Which children should be treated? How much
medication should they receive? How long should AEDs be used?
Doctors' views on AEDs have changed. Several decades ago, many
doctors believed that seizures must be stopped at all costs and that, once
stopped, medications should be continued for prolonged periods or
indefinitely. This outdated approach reflected an overly pessimistic
outlook on life with epilepsy. The risks of seizures were overestimated,
and medications' side effects were underestimated. Issues such as the
quality of life, or how patients felt about seizures and side effects, were
rarely considered, and the natural course of epilepsy was poorly understood. Greater understanding has led to a better balance of seizure
control and AED use.

Stopping AEDs

Most children who remain seizure-free while taking medications for
1 or 2 years can safely have their medications slowly tapered by their
doctors and eventually discontinued. Most of these children will not
have another seizure. The current trend is toward discontinuing AEDs

Table 19.1. Risk Factors for Predicting Recurrent Seizure in Children				
	EEG: no epileptiform discharges		EEG: epileptiform discharges	
Diagnosis	Neuro exam, normal	Neuro exam, abnormal	Neuro exam, normal	Neuro exam, abnormal
Tonic-clonic	30%	51%	47%	73%
Simple partial	50%	75%	71%	92%
Complex partial	58%	83%	77%	96%

Source: Camfield PR et al., Neurology 1985;35:1657–1660.

earlier rather than later because the chances of staying seizure-free after 1 or 2 years are similar to those after 4 years. Among children who remain seizure-free while taking AEDs for 2 years, approximately 65% will remain seizure-free after the medication is stopped.

The chance that a specific child will remain seizure-free if medications are stopped cannot be predicted with accuracy. Table 19.1 shows some factors associated with the risk of having a seizure after AEDs are stopped in seizure-free children. Favorable signs for remaining seizure-free include the lack of an identifiable cause for epilepsy, normal development and neurological function, the absence of epilepsy waves on the EEG, and seizures that were easily controlled with medication. When all of these conditions are met, the child has an excellent chance to remain seizure-free off AEDs.

No matter how good the odds, however, there is a chance that the seizures will recur, and no matter how bad the odds, there is a chance that they will not. Many cases fall between the extremes, making the decision more difficult. As a general rule, it is usually worthwhile to attempt to discontinue the medication after 2 years of seizure-freedom. When the child has two or more risk factors for seizure recurrence (first seizure after 12 years of age, neurologic or intellectual disabilities, or complex partial seizures), it may be reasonable to continue AEDs until the child has been seizure-free for 3 or 4 years before attempting to withdraw them.

Signs indicating a greater chance of seizure recurrence off AEDs are a progressive brain disorder or brain damage such as a birth injury; viral infection of the brain; head injury, developmental delay, mental retardation, or other neurologic abnormalities; the presence of epilepsy waves or moderate to severe slowing on the EEG; and seizures that were not easily controlled with AEDs. When all of these factors are present, the chance of seizures recurring after medication is stopped is 50% or more. These are *average* risks, however, which cannot easily be applied to a particular individual.

Some times are better than others for stopping AEDs. For example, a girl who is on a gymnastics team and who does difficult dismounts on the uneven parallel bars probably should not begin tapering medications shortly before the gymnastic season. Summer camp, when the child will be swimming and boating, presents a similar situation. For those approaching driving age, consider a trial off AEDs at least 6–12 months before they are eligible for a license.

When all of these risks are considered, some parents and children may ask, "Why not simply continue to take the drugs? They don't seem to be doing any harm." If there is a moderate to high risk of seizure recurrence, and the medications have few side effects, the risks of stopping the drug may outweigh the benefits.

Risks of Stopping Medication

I was frightened when the doctor recommended that we take Katie off the Tegretol. Of course I wanted her off all medications, but even more I wanted her seizure-free. We lowered the medication slowly. I slept poorly for months, thinking that any noise in the house was a seizure. She's been off medication for 3 years, and has had no seizures.

The greatest danger of stopping AEDs is the risk of recurrent seizures. If the medications are stopped abruptly, a recurrent seizure might be more severe or prolonged than the previous seizures.

Discontinuation of an AED can cause a withdrawal reaction. The rapid withdrawal of barbiturates (phenobarbital and primidone) or benzodiazepines (clonazepam, clorazepate, diazepam, lorazepam, and clobazam) carries the highest risk of a seizure or unpleasant symptoms such as anxiety, irritability, a racing heart, difficulty sleeping, sweating, and abdominal pain. Withdrawal symptoms are reduced or eliminated when the dosage is lowered very slowly. Rapid discontinuation of any

Table 19.2. Tips on Discontinuing Antiepileptic Drugs

- First-aid management should be reviewed with the child, the parents, and other caregivers.

- The usual medication should be kept on hand in case the child's seizures recur.

- If a seizure occurs, it may be appropriate to give the child a single dose of medication before contacting the doctor.

- If status epilepticus is a concern or access to medical care is a problem, parents should be taught how to administer diazepam (Diastat) rectally or buccal midazolam when a seizure lasts longer than 5 minutes.

- A child who has a recurrent seizure is expected to be depressed, upset, or angry, but if the mood change persists longer than a week, a visit to the doctor is recommended.

- It may be comforting to use an intercom system between the parent's and child's bedrooms or an alerting device, such as the one made by Fisher-Price and costing less than $50, at bedtime or when the child is asleep in case of a seizure recurrence. For a greater level of monitoring, a device can detect movement (detector under mattress) and signal parents in their room, although a certain amount movement during the seizure is needed to activate the device (easylinkuk.co.uk; ~$350).

AED can be dangerous and cause status epilepticus and should only be done under a doctor's supervision.

When an AED is tapered or withdrawn, seizures may occur because the drug was needed to control them. Depending on the type and severity of the seizures, the AED(s) may need to be restarted, although the child may remain seizure-free at a lower dosage than before. Differentiating this type of seizure recurrence from a withdrawal seizure is important, because withdrawal seizures can be managed by a temporary increase in the dosage followed by more gradual tapering.

If AEDs are stopped, the child, family, and school need to be prepared for a possible seizure. During the tapering and for at least 3–6 months after stopping the medications, the child's risk of a seizure is somewhat higher than usual, and simple precautions should be taken, (see Table 19.2). The child should not swim without close supervision or climb to high places. Three quarters of seizure relapses occur within 1 year of stopping the medication.

If a seizure recurs after a period of freedom from seizures, it is an emotional setback for both the child and the family. Discuss the possibility. When people are aware that something is possible, they can handle it better if it happens. Although children (and parents!) often will privately worry about a possible seizure, their fear diminishes with time.

A rare consequence of discontinuing the medication is the reemergence of difficult-to-control seizures or the development of intolerance to an AED that was previously well tolerated. Luckily, this is very uncommon.

Benefits of Stopping Medication

In the best of all worlds, when the medications are stopped, seizures will not recur and the child will feel better and will have improved school performance and behavior. When a child takes a medicine for more than 1–2 years, it can be difficult to estimate the effect that the drug has on the child's behavior. This is particularly true if the dosage was gradually increased over a long period. In many cases, although the medication was thought to have no side effects, the child's alertness, ability to concentrate, memory, ability to reason, and behavioral problems such as irritability and hyperactivity improve after the medication is stopped. Some AEDs, however, such as carbamazepine, lamotrigine, and valproate, can have positive effects on a child's mood and behavior, and occasionally their discontinuation is associated with increased behavioral problems.

Long-Term Treatment

Although most forms of childhood epilepsy are outgrown, some forms are associated with a high risk of recurrent seizures if the medications are stopped. If the EEG shows abundant epilepsy waves or epilepsy waves arising from multiple regions of the brain, the risk of seizures after stopping medications is high. Juvenile myoclonic epilepsy, for example, is associated with a high rate of seizure recurrence after AEDs are stopped. This epilepsy disorder varies dramatically in its severity, however, and some children have only mild myoclonic jerks a few hours after awakening. For them, stopping the medication may be reasonable. In Lennox-Gastaut syndrome, the seizures are severe and difficult to control. If control is achieved, it is usually wise to continue the medication or possibly reduce the dosage of the medication slightly.

20 | Intellectual and Behavioral Development

Most children with epilepsy are developmentally normal. However, children who have frequent or severe seizures that remain uncontrolled, are treated with large amounts of AEDs, or have other brain disorders often experience some developmental delays. If development is delayed, the pediatric neurologist or developmental pediatrician should evaluate the cause of the delay and what it may mean for the future. It is difficult for doctors to accurately predict the child's future development. It can be difficult to determine the contributing roles of physical brain abnormality, seizures, or medications in delayed development. All of these factors can be involved to varying degrees.

The pace or slope of developmental progress is relative. Children with severe cerebral palsy or mental retardation develop! The rate may be slow, the process laborious, but the gains are no less meaningful and exciting. In rare cases of degenerative disorders, development can regress. Some children with epilepsy may lose some milestones previously attained, but the loss is often temporary.

> JJ developed tonic-clonic seizures without fever at age 8 months. He was started on phenobarbital and did well for several months. Then tonic-clonic and myoclonic seizures developed and continued despite high dosages of phenobarbital and other drugs. At age 14 months, his development stopped. The MRI revealed cortical dysplasia (abnormal organization of the brain). The pediatric neurologist started him on clonazepam, and the seizures lessened, but within 2 weeks his walking became unsteady. A diagnosis of a degenerative disorder was incorrectly made, and a dismal prognosis was described to the child's mother. Another neurologist tapered him off of clonazepam and he again walked normally. JJ, now 8 years old, takes no medications, and has been seizure-free for more than 4 years. His motor skills are excellent.

Effects of Seizures and AEDs on Mental Functions

Single seizures do not permanently impair intellectual or behavioral functions. The long-term effects of recurrent seizures are not fully understood and vary for different children. Mild seizures, such as absence and simple partial seizures, even when recurrent over years, are not known to cause permanent problems. Yet, even here there is evidence that such children have higher rates of academic and social problems than other children. Children with frequent complex partial seizures may have memory impairment and behavioral disorders, but it is not proven that the seizures cause these problems. Many have structural abnormalities in brain areas that control memory or emotion, and these problems can cause cognitive and behavioral difficulties.

Frequent or prolonged tonic-clonic seizures are associated with lower scores on intelligence and memory, suggesting that these seizures can be harmful. Also, a large number of lifetime tonic-clonic seizures or status epilepticus are associated with impaired mental function. However, other brain disorders are often present, and the intellectual problems can be caused by the underlying brain disorder as well as recurrent seizures, head injury, AEDs, and psychosocial factors. Teasing out the effects of these factors in clinical studies and individual patients is difficult. Any of these factors can predominate in causing a problem in a specific child. However, the effect of recurrent complex partial and tonic-clonic seizures has probably been underestimated. Parents often overestimate the negative effects of AEDs.

AEDs can impair intellectual performance and cause behavioral problems. However, among the primary AEDs used at standard doses (see Table 12.1), these effects are usually slight. In studies comparing children's cognitive (intellectual) functions before and after the discontinuation of AEDs, cognitive functions were not improved or only slightly improved off the drugs. However, the cognitive and behavioral effects of AEDs are often dose-related. Therefore, children on high AED dosages are more likely to suffer side effects. Also, although group averages may show no statistical difference, some individuals may experience disabling problems, even at low doses.

The first pediatric neurologist told me that phenobarbital was like water, that we would never know that Brenda was on it. He was wrong. She became cranky, hyperactive, slept poorly- she was a different child. We were told this would pass, but it only seemed to get worse as time went on. We lost our child. If we had to choose, we would take the seizures ever side effect. A second opinion changed her to Tegretol. We have our daughter back.

Sally was just starting to speak; she had at least 12 words and was such a bright girl. The Topamax really shut down her speech. On the lower dose it slowed down and became more effortful and as we pushed it up, she stopped speaking. Five days off the Topamax she was back.

As the dosage and blood levels of AED increase, side effects also increase. Excessive drowsiness and need for sleep, slowed thinking and movement, decreased initiative and motivation, memory lapses, and other cognitive deficits become more pronounced with higher blood levels. AED combinations are also more likely to cause cognitive problems, as well as other adverse effects. When high doses or combinations of AED are used, there must be a careful balance between the positive and negative effects.

No seizures, no side effects: in some cases, this goal cannot be attained, and the effects of the seizures must be weighed against AED side effects. For example, the doctor probably would not choose to increase the dosage to the point of sedation or emotional and intellectual dulling to reduce complex partial seizures from three to two a month. Medicine side effects would be present, in varying degrees, throughout each day of the child's life, whereas a complex partial seizure last minutes.

Difficult decisions about the use of AEDs come when the side effects are subtle and intermittent. A description of the child's behavior, based on the parent's observations and supplemented by reports from teachers and others is invaluable to the doctor. Carefully document side effects and their relation to when medications are taken. Both side effects and seizures can often be reduced by changes in the timing of AED doses. For example, the medication can be given after meals to minimize peak side effects caused by rapid absorption of the drug. In other cases, more frequent but smaller doses can help to maintain more steady blood levels of the drug, thereby reducing side effects and improving seizure control. When side effects are bothersome in the daytime, or seizures are most likely to occur during sleep or shortly after awakening, the bedtime or after-dinner dose can be increased and the daytime doses decreased. Midday doses during should be avoided, if possible, so that the child does not have to go to the school nurse.

When a child has taken AEDs for years, it may be difficult to distinguish effects of medication from "who the child is." Even if the child has been seizure-free for years and can understand the question, "Does the medication make you tired or cause any other problems?," they may not be able to remember what it was like to be off medications and, therefore, cannot really answer. Lowering, discontinuing, or switching medications may be the only way to find out.

Building Self-Esteem in Children with Epilepsy

> It seems strange that it took a social worker at the epilepsy center to make me realize what I had been doing. Doing everything for Tricia was making her more dependent on me—making her bed, helping her dress, clearing her dishes, staying within a few feet in case she had a seizure—all because I love her. I never thought she could put her own sneakers on until she did it at the hospital. It is hard to let go, but exciting.

Of all the things that parents can give children, the opportunity to develop self-esteem and self-confidence may be most important. For children to develop, learn, and interact at school and to grow successfully toward independence and adulthood, they must have a strong and positive sense of self. Building self-esteem requires a parent to be patient, to use educational discipline, to provide opportunities for children to do things independently, and to praise them for their initiatives and progress.

The parents of a child with epilepsy must first maintain their own self-esteem (see Chapter 27). Having a child with an illness, especially one that has been associated with negative attitudes, is difficult. Even very young children can sense their parents' feelings.

Parents must emphasize the positive and minimize the negative. Focus on the things the child can do and build on those achievements. Negative messages can limit self-esteem and motivation. Parents must not show their frustration at what the child cannot do or compare their child negatively with siblings or other children. Talking about "the problem" in front of the child is not good. This is not to say that parents should not discuss the epilepsy in a supportive fashion, but they should not focus on the child as a problem. The child's condition must not be used as an excuse for limiting his or her participation in activities such as school clubs or scouts, as this will send the message to the child that the parents do not have confidence in him or her. Supportive resources are available (see Appendix D).

Encouraging Personal Responsibility

Children with and without epilepsy can understand epilepsy. Children should be told about the disorder in words they can understand—why taking medication on time is important, why tests are done, and why certain activities may have to be restricted. Children usually understand more than adults think they do.

If possible, a child should know the name of his or her medication, the color of the pill, the dosage, and the medication schedule. Although an attentive parent can do everything and allow the child to become a passive participant in his or her care, this should be resisted. Foster trust and knowledge, not disability.

Avoiding Overprotectiveness

There is a fine line between healthy caution and overprotection. Parents have a strong and natural tendency to direct their children's behavior. They want them to do the things they think are right and avoid things they consider wrong or dangerous. For children with epilepsy, this tendency may become exaggerated, and parents may drift into being overprotective. They are often unaware of their directive behavior, or fiercely defend it. Doing everything for children and restricting their exposure to the usual challenges of childhood takes away independence, slows their social growth, and lowers their self-esteem.

Overprotectiveness can take many forms. In the extreme form, older children may never be told they have epilepsy; they are told their medications are "vitamins" or simply not told anything. Some children and young adults are largely confined to their houses because of parental fear that they could of injury if they go out. Mild overprotectiveness is much more common.

Children usually survive their parents. Most children will become independent long before their parents are gone. However, many children with severe epilepsy and neurologic disorders remain dependent and will require some degree of supportive care throughout their lives. Parents must plan ahead of time for such a child eventually to live in some type of supportive environment, such as a residential home or "independent living center."

Encouraging Social Contacts

One of the most important parts of childhood is learning to relate, play, disagree, share, make friendships, and grow together—to socialize. The greatest cost of overprotection and isolation may be limited social contacts. No matter how loving and giving parents are, they can never replace the joys and lessons that children bring to each other. Although children can be cruel, parents must move beyond the fears of possible problems. Children need other children.

Parents should encourage their child's participation in activities with other children. These activities can range from play groups and play dates to extracurricular activities such as sports, dancing, singing, or crafts and, for older children, independently playing with other children after school and on weekends. Emphasize inclusion, not exclusion. Although the parents may believe some activities are unsafe, special precautions, including closer supervision, can be used to make these activities safer.

Children with epilepsy may benefit from meeting, talking, and playing with other children who have epilepsy. Epilepsy.com provides a list of summer camps (www.epilepsy.com/info/family_camplist.html). For a child to learn that he or she is not alone can be enormously comforting. If an area has no groups for children with epilepsy, a motivated parent can start one.

Using Educational Discipline

Susie has always been impossible. She does what she wants, when she wants. Nothing worked—taking away her favorite toys or foods, sending her up to her room, or raising my voice. We wanted to give up. Then a friend with a child who has cerebral palsy and hyperactivity told me that we were inconsistent, often giving in to her tantrums. We reacted to Susie with frustration, never really understanding her needs. It took a lot of hard work. Before Susie could change, we had to change. Now Susie's favorite book is *Clifford's Manners* (see Appendix D).

Some parents of children with epilepsy overindulge them and ignore bad behaviors as a way of "making up" for the epilepsy or because they fear that sterner punishment will cause more seizures. Although seizures can occasionally be brought on by emotional stress, there is no evidence that they are caused by educational discipline. Educational discipline means explaining why the child's behavior was wrong and withholding something the child desires or using the technique of "time out," in which, for example, the child must go to the corner of the room and stand quietly for a minute because of bad behavior. An undisciplined child can face serious problems in learning to socialize with other children, to behave and learn at school, and to grow up to be an independent adult. Ultimately, these problems will lead to much greater stress.

Behavioral Problems

Behavioral problems can occur around the time of a seizure of apart from seizures. This section looks at problems that are special but not unique for children with epilepsy: learning disorders, difficulty with concentration (attention deficit), hyperactivity, and language and cognitive impairments, as well as anxiety, irritability, aggressive verbal or physical behavior, depression, mood swings, poor social skills, lack of motivation and energy, and inability to plan and organize behavior.

Learning Disorders

Children with learning disorders have a discrepancy between intellectual level and academic achievement; that is, intelligence outpaces achievement. Neurologic disorders such as epilepsy can cause learning disorders, although most children with epilepsy do not have learning disorders.

Learning requires a complicated series of brain processes. The absorption process requires paying attention and perceiving (seeing and hearing the material). The memory process requires actively comparing the newly acquired information with previously learned information and recalling it when necessary. These are but a few of the many complex steps in the process of learning.

The most extensively studied learning disorder is dyslexia, a developmental reading disorder. The cause is not understood, but the functions of the left temporal and parietal lobes, areas critical for reading and language comprehension, are implicated. Seizures can affect these areas. However, reading can be impaired by many kinds of problems. Children who cannot focus their attention for more than a few seconds can have secondary reading problems. Visual problems affecting the eyes or the brain processing of visual information can impair reading. Reading can also be disrupted by right (nonlanguage) hemisphere disorders that impair visual attention.

Other learning problems effect learning arithmetic, spoken information, visual information other than reading, relating visual information to movement components (visuomotor disorders), or relating objects in space (disorders of visuospatial analysis). Other children have difficulty understanding social rules and emotionally relating to peers or adults.

When a learning disability is suspected, the child should be evaluated by a school psychologist, neuropsychologist, or child study team. Such services can be requested through the child's school (see Chapter 21). The evaluation can often identify the type of and cause of a learning disorder. Testing should be comprehensive to avoid misdiagnosis and to ensure proper placement and therapies.

Attention Deficit Disorder

Attention is the cornerstone on which intellectual functions rest. If we do not pay attention, we cannot efficiently understand, learn, or remember. Attentional filtering prevents our minds from becoming overwhelmed by the bombardment of images and sensations from our mind, body, and environment. The attentional filtering system develops in children around the time that fine movement control and ability to learn abstract mathematic relationships also develop. A 3-year-old simply cannot sit quietly for 3 hours and read.

Attention deficit disorder (ADD) is a common problem in school-children and is characterized by the inability to maintain attention, poor concentration, distractibility, and impulsivity. These problems exceed the normal behavior for the child's age and interfere with learning. They are usually noticed by teachers and parents. ADD usually begins before the age of 5 years and is more common in boys. Hyperactivity and ADD often co-exist in the same child. The two disorders are separate, however, and one may occur without the other. ADD refers to cognitive behavior, whereas hyperactivity refers to motor behavior. Children with epilepsy have higher incidences of both ADD and hyperactivity. In some children with epilepsy, the attentional and hyperactivity problem is related to the underlying neurologic problem.

The cause of ADD is unknown. Parents of some children report that consumption of sugar "sets them off," reducing their attention span. Medical studies, however, have generally not found dietary restrictions to be effective, other than the possibility that eliminating foods with colorings and additives may improve 5–10% of cases. ADD may be a disorder of brain maturity or a chemical imbalance. Most children outgrow their ADD, although many continue to have problems in adolescence and adulthood.

Medications can cause or accentuate attentional problems. Any drug that makes a person tired can impair attention. Barbiturates and benzo-diazepines can cause hyperactivity and impair attention. If attentional problems develop after a drug is started or the dosage is increased, inform the doctor. The problem may lessen within weeks or a few months; in other cases, the dosage must be reduced or the medication changed.

When ADD causes learning or social problems, medical therapy may be helpful. Behavioral modification is of limited benefit and less effective than medication for ADD. The drugs used to treat ADD include stimulants and atomoxetine (Strattera). In children with ADD, stimu-lants paradoxically lead to a more relaxed and focused state of mind. The most commonly used stimulants are methylphenidate (Ritalin, Concerta, Metadate) and amphetamines (Adderal, Dexedrine). They can be used safely in children for prolonged periods, but must be carefully supervised by a doctor. Side effects include decreased appetite and weight loss, stomach discomfort, difficulty sleeping, depression, and irritability. Long-term use may slightly decrease growth. As the child grows older, gradual reduction of the ADD medications should be considered, because the disorder is often outgrown.

In the vast majority of children with epilepsy, stimulant drugs can be used safely. Insomnia, a potential side effect, may increase seizure activity. Methylphenidate can occasionally exacerbate seizures, especially in children whose seizures are not fully controlled by AEDs. When ADD is diagnosed, the majority of children with epilepsy can experience improved attention with no worsening of seizure control on a stimulant. Many children do not take stimulants on weekends and vacations.

Amotoxetine is a nonstimulant alternative to treat ADD and hyperactivity. It can be safely used in epilepsy patients. It has fewer side effects (does not suppress appetite or growth and does not cause insomnia), but many find it less effective than stimulants.

Impulsivity can affect a child's social relations and academic achievements. Impulsivity is characterized by a tendency to act automatically in response to environmental stimuli, without considering the consequences of the actions. The ability to reflect on one's actions and consider long-term effects is only fully achieved in adulthood. Stimulants, amotoxetine, and clonidine (Catapress) can reduce impulsivity. Clonidine can cause sedation but does not worsen seizure control.

Hyperactivity

Children are much more physically active than adults. In some children, excessive movement, or hyperactivity, causes problems. The increased activity may take several forms, such as excessive fidgeting, an inability to stay seated for more than a minute, and running around endlessly. Hyperactivity causes problems because it prevents the child, usually a boy, from staying in one place and can disrupt the classroom and home.

Hyperactivity is slightly more common among children with epilepsy. It is also more common among children with tic disorders and mental handicap. The drugs that can improve ADD can also treat hyperactivity.

Severe Language, Cognitive, and Behavioral Impairments

Some children with epilepsy have severe language and cognitive impairments. Social and behavioral problems may further impair their intellectual development, because socializing is the primary process by which children obtain language skills. Similarly, language impairment can severely hinder social play. Most children react positively to a voice or smile, but to many children with severe developmental disabilities such as autism, these sounds and gestures can be threatening and confusing. Their reactions to stimuli are inappropriate, unpredictable, and sometimes destructive.

Some children may only communicate *on their own terms*. Fortunately, behavior management techniques are available to change the child's avoidance patterns and create new patterns of interaction, which can provide the child with a base of trust in our complicated world (see Appendix D). Applied behavioral analysis (ABA) is a technique that incorporates a comprehensive but individual plan to increase skills and decrease unwanted behaviors. In many children with developmental delay, psychiatric disorders must be assessed and treated.

21 | Telling Children and Others About Epilepsy

Epilepsy was once shrouded in secrecy. The word, like "cancer" or "leprosy," evoked fear and isolation. Those days are largely gone. The more the word "epilepsy" is used, the more children and adults understand epilepsy, and the more an openness surrounds it, the more the secrecy and fear will disappear.

Telling Children About Epilepsy

Children should be told about epilepsy. I recently met a woman who was never told about her disorder, which began when she was 6. She finally went to a library at age 20 to research her symptoms and recognized that she had been treated for epilepsy but was never told about it. She was furious at her parents and doctors.

When and how much do you tell a child about epilepsy? The child must not be overwhelmed with words and ideas that are either incomprehensible or frightening, but "protecting" the child by withholding the truth can be the worst choice. In general, children under 3 years of age do not need to be told anything. After the age of 3, children can usually understand if epilepsy is explained in simple language without the use of medical words. Parents need to keep it simple and be positive about the problem.

The book *Lee, the Rabbit with Epilepsy* by Deborah Moss is a brightly illustrated book for young children. It describes how the rabbit with epilepsy visits the doctor, takes medication, and, most importantly, continues to enjoy life.

Telling Others Who Need to Know

Anyone who is teaching, caring for, or closely associated with a child with epilepsy should know about the child's disorder. If someone responsible for a child's health or safety doesn't know that the child has epilepsy, avoidable problems can occur.

In some cultures, parents may be especially reluctant to discuss their child's epilepsy. These are often the same cultures in which there are strong concerns about epilepsy and marriage. For example, some members of the Asian and Orthodox Jewish communities have strong reservations about disclosing the presence of epilepsy in a family member. This attitude is mostly based on concerns regarding stigma and discrimination. However, a child's health should take precedence over other concerns.

Relatives

Relatives can be the most supportive and helpful people in the world or the most difficult. As a general rule, relatives should be told about a child's epilepsy. Who and how much to tell should depend on whether or not the relatives are likely to be alone with the child and how they may react. Practically speaking, however, if one relative has been told, they have all been told! A potential problem with relatives is that they love to give advice. Advice is often helpful, but the primary caregivers (usually the parents) must do what they feel is best for the child. As the child gets older, he or she should begin to assume some of this responsibility.

School Nurses, Teachers, and Classmates

School is a major part of the child's day. If the child has daytime seizures, school nurses and teachers should be told about the child's epilepsy. The school nurse is the child's advocate in the school and a resource for teachers who need information. The school nurse is most likely to be called on if the child has a seizure or experiences medication side effects. The nurse should know the child's seizure type(s), the medications, and parent's and doctor's telephone numbers. The school nurse may confer with the gym teacher or sports coach to discuss possible precautions during some activities.

The teacher should know the type of seizures the child has and what they look like. Teachers who are not familiar with epilepsy or with the child's seizure type can be given a pamphlet, video, or website (epilepsy.com) telling them about how to recognize seizures, first aid for seizures, and side effects of medications.

If daytime seizures are frequent, discuss the disorder with the rest of the children in the class. Time can be set aside to discuss epilepsy and the child's seizures. By discussing it openly, the children can be educated and a sense of community is fostered. A staff member from the local Epilepsy Foundation or an epilepsy center may conduct an educational program for the child's classmates or the school. These forums can help in shift the other children's perspective from fear and teasing to respect and friendship.

The Child's Friends and Their Parents

> Pete just wants to be one of the kids. He has overcome a learning disability and is now in mainstream classes and doing well. He has a few good friends and loves basketball. Although his seizures are now well controlled, he doesn't want anyone at school to know about his epilepsy. We have tried to convince him to tell his close friends, but he refuses.

Children with epilepsy should be encouraged to pursue friendships and social activities, which are essential for self-esteem and future success. The decision to tell a friend about epilepsy is often difficult. Children can be insensitive. In addition, if the friend's parents are uninformed about epilepsy, they may fear for their child's safety or "psychological trauma" if they witness a seizure.

The child's friends and their parents should be told about the child's epilepsy, but it should not just be casually mentioned. It may be a good idea for the young person to discuss the epilepsy with his or her close friends and for the parent to discuss the disorder one-on-one with the friends' parents. The discussion should explain the type of seizures, their frequency, how the seizures affect the child, and what to do in case a seizure occurs. Most important, they need to know that epilepsy is just another episodic medical problem, like asthma, which affects otherwise healthy, active children. The other children and their parents also should be given a chance to ask questions.

The need to conform and to belong to a group makes many adolescents want to hide their epilepsy. Therefore, whether to tell their friends about epilepsy can be a difficult decision. *The adolescent must always be involved in the decision to reveal his or her disorder–whom to tell, how to tell, and how much to tell.*

Babysitters

Babysitters allow parents to have some independence from their children. Babysitters who are educated about the disorder can care for children with epilepsy. Although parents are right in thinking that no one will watch and care for their children the way they do, mature and responsible babysitters can do a very good job. Children also need to learn that their parents cannot be there every minute.

Babysitters should be told that a child has epilepsy before they agree to watch the child. Because babysitters are left alone with the child, they should have basic knowledge about epilepsy and first aid. They should be reassured that dangerous situations and emergencies are extremely uncommon, but they must be prepared. They should know the type of seizures, medication dosage, where the medication is stored, and the telephone numbers of those to call in an emergency, including the doctor's number. For children with seizures associated with incontinence, keeping a change of clothing on hand for the child (and the babysitter) can be helpful.

The Dentist and Orthodontist

Although children with epilepsy rarely require special attention during dental procedures, dentists should be made aware of the child's seizure disorder. For children with frequent seizures, a low dose of a benzodiaze-pine, such as lorazepam, may be helpful before dental procedures. Children with epilepsy who are taking medications that affect gum growth should receive regular dental care and should be taught to brush with care and, when old enough, to use dental floss.

Children with severe epilepsy, cerebral palsy, or associated neurological disorders may require general anesthesia for major dental work. Before such procedures, it may be helpful for the dentist and doctor to discuss the medications and precautions. Finally, the orthodontist should know that the child has epilepsy because special precautions may be needed when braces are fitted.

22 | Family Life, Social Life, and Physical Activities

The effects of epilepsy on children's behavioral, intellectual, and social development are extremely variable. Most children with epilepsy lead normal lives and have few or no restrictions on social or physical activities. For some children, seizures and AED side effects cause many difficulties. Other children have additional medical and neurologic problems.

Family and Social Life

A child's illness complicates the challenges of family life. The epilepsy of a child with minor seizures that are fully controlled should not unduly affect the family. But when a child's seizures are frequent or severe, or when the child also has other physical or neurologic disorders, family life is always affected. All relationships in the family are changed—between parents, parent–child, siblings, and the child with epilepsy.

The child with epilepsy has special needs, but so do his or her siblings. As their age and maturity permit, siblings should be educated about epilepsy. Because the child with epilepsy will draw time and attention like a magnet, parents must make special time for their other children.

Getting on with Life

> Initially, Jim and I were so consumed by Anthony's epilepsy that nothing else seemed to matter. Between the seizures, medications, doctor visits, tests, meetings with teachers, and our jobs, there was no time for anything else. It took us 6 months or so, but we have finally realized that life goes on for Anthony, for his older brother Paul, and for us. We do special things with Paul to let him know how much we love him. We also have our parents come every few months to spend the weekend with the kids so that we can just get away.

Once the child's epilepsy has been diagnosed, treatment has begun, and some time has passed for understanding and accepting the disorder, it is time for the parents to get on with their lives. In the cases of moderate severity, with intermittent seizures and medication side effects and social and academic issues, resuming a full life is a challenge. In the most serious cases it may seem impossible, but it is not.

Parents must accept the disorder and the associated disorders for what they are and understand the needs of the child with epilepsy and their other children, as well as their own needs and those of their partner-find the best care for their child, decide how they want to live their lives, and then believe that they can do it. Some parents feel as if they are swept up in a current. That is true for everyone at the beginning. Parents cannot passively ride the current, however, or they will find themselves in a place they do not want to be. They must determine the direction.

Unfortunately, divorce is much more common among parents who have children with developmental disabilities than among couples in general. Early recognition of the additional stress and open communication is critical.

Counseling

> I thought that Jake told us everything. It seemed like he was doing great. We never suspected that things were bothering him—the epilepsy, pressure to get good grades, and other kids in his school. It was building up inside for a while. When the school called to ask how he was doing, we realized that he had been missing classes for a while, telling the teachers he had seizures. It was all too much for him. The counselor was a godsend. Jake needs us, but he also needs someone else.

Parents, siblings, grandparents, and teachers provide children with role models, advice, guidance, and support. They provide a nurturing environment and a positive outlook, but usually none of them has epilepsy. Despite their best intentions and loving support, they often fail to ask, "How do you feel about having epilepsy?" "How do you think other kids react to you because you have epilepsy?" "Do you understand what the doctor said?" "What are your greatest fears?"

Most children with epilepsy do not require formal counseling, but all of them require education about the disorder and help in learning to adjust to it. A counselor can provide the outside perspective that is often lacking. Parental concern may be misdirected into telling the child how to feel and how to act. Although all parents feel that they know what is best for their children, it can be difficult to determine what is truly best. A dialogue is often much more helpful than an "answer." A counselor can help "open" the part of the child that epilepsy can hide. The essence of counseling is to provide understanding and help the person cope with the medical and social impact of the disorder. Counseling can help the child and the entire family.

Friendships

Children with epilepsy should be encouraged to pursue friendships and social activities like other children. Perhaps the most negative effect of epilepsy on children is the isolation and rejection that may accompany the disorder, often unnecessarily. A child must be given independence to pursue healthy friendships. Parents may face conflicting desires: encourage play with other children but protect the child from danger. Physical injury can be caused by seizures, but the emotional trauma of isolation is probably more painful and more long-lasting.

Many parents would like their child to be more active in friendships and social activities but find that the child fears rejection or that his or her opportunities are limited. The social activities of some children are limited by other neurological and emotional disorders. For these children, community programs and networking between parents can be helpful.

Going to Camp

All children with epilepsy can enjoy camp. Those with well-controlled or occasional seizures can attend a regular camp. The range of activities and precautions must be individually specified, but these children can usually enjoy a very full and active camp experience. Children with frequent seizures, or children who have never met another child with epilepsy, may benefit from going to a camp with other children who have epilepsy. Epilepsy.com (epilepsy.com/info/family_summercamp.html) and the local Epilepsy Foundation can provide information about these camps. Scholarships may be available from organizations such as Finding a Cure for Epilepsy and Seizures (FACES; med.nyu.edu/faces).

Some camps specialize in programs for children with severe epilepsy, cerebral palsy, or emotional disorders. They provide a wonderful social opportunity for the children and an important respite for parents.

Physical Activities and Sports

The balance between a child's safety and the ability to enjoy a full range of activities is tested when it comes to recommendations regarding sports and other physical activities. Because epilepsy affects each person differently, the approach must be individualized. The type and frequency of the seizures, the medication and its side effects, the child's ability to follow instructions and act responsibly, and the nature and supervision of the activity must all be considered.

Common sense should guide these decisions. The goals should be both safety and a lifestyle that is as normal as possible. No activity is completely safe. Making safety the exclusive concern will unnecessarily limit the child's activities. Restriction and isolation foster low self-esteem and emphasize the disability. Nevertheless, certain activities can be dangerous and safety concerns require that these activities be forbidden or carefully supervised. Children with epilepsy should pursue as full a range of activity as reasonable.

The type of seizures and their frequency are critical in determining which activities are safe. Children whose motor control or consciousness is impaired during seizures are at higher risk for injuries. Children who have uncontrolled, frequent seizures should know that certain activities are restricted. For example, they should not swim alone (in fact, *no* child should swim alone), or play on high bars or climb ropes without a proper mat and supervision. Other activities, such as riding a bicycle in traffic, should be forbidden. However, bicycling may be permitted in safer settings. If a child's seizures are more common at certain times (within 2 hours of awakening, for example), activities can be scheduled when seizures are less likely to occur.

Seizures are only rarely provoked by exercise, especially in hot weather, but when this pattern is identified, physical exertion should be limited. However, exercise is still possible, but the level of exertion should be monitored and rest periods and hydration may help prevent seizures.

Children with epilepsy should be encouraged to participate in group and competitive sports, such as community sports, Little League baseball, and school sports. These activities are usually well supervised and require appropriate safety gear.

Serious injuries in children with epilepsy are uncommon and rarely occur during participation in sports. Bathrooms can be much more dangerous to children with epilepsy than playing soccer or ice skating.

Stair Climbing

Our world is filled with stairs. For the vast majority of children with epilepsy, stairs should not be barriers to getting around. However, seizures that impair motor control or consciousness can cause serious injuries if they occur while the child is on a staircase. If a child has an aura, or warning, before a seizure, he or she may be able to sit down until the seizure is over. If the child has frequent seizures that cause falling, it is not unreasonable to have him or her use elevators, not stairs.

Bathing

Children with uncontrolled seizures should not bathe in a tub unsupervised. Such children should take tub baths only when they can be supervised. As children get older, however, they need privacy, and this means that they must take showers. Bathroom doors should never be locked.

Swimming and Water Sports

Swimming poses special dangers for children with epilepsy, but no matter how severe or frequent the epilepsy, a child can enjoy the water. A parent can hold a child in a shallow pool with little risk, for instance. If the child's seizures are well controlled, swimming should be encouraged, although at least one person who knows the child has epilepsy and who knows basic lifesaving must be nearby.

The most difficult decisions about swimming arise when children have occasional seizures that impair motor control or consciousness. These children can swim with close supervision. There should be a lifeguard who is responsible and aware of the child's disorder. When possible, another child in the pool can be the buddy. Unfortunately, lifeguards are often adolescents who may be easily distracted. The lifeguards should know that they *must* keep their eyes on the pool while the child is swimming. The buddy system, used by many camps for young children who swim (and by adult scuba divers), is another precaution to ensure a child's safety.

Swimming in a lake, bay, or ocean is much more dangerous than swimming in a pool. A person swimming in open waters can disappear in seconds and be impossible to locate quickly. Therefore, extreme caution must be exercised when a child with epilepsy, especially one with poorly controlled seizures, swims in open waters. Lifejackets are recommended in this setting.

Older children with well-controlled seizures can snorkel and may even scuba dive. Children with uncontrolled seizures that impair consciousness or motor control should not scuba dive and should only snorkel in relatively calm water, very close to someone who has lifesaving skills.

Bicycling

Bicycles on or near the street can cause a serious potential danger for a child with epilepsy. Even if a parent rides just behind the child on the sidewalk, during a complex partial seizure the child may suddenly veer off into the street. Despite the dangers, children with epilepsy can learn to ride and enjoy bicycles. If the seizures are under control or do not impair motor control or consciousness, bicycle riding should be unrestricted. When the seizures pose a danger, bicycles can be ridden in a park or other safe areas.

Stationary bicycles for exercise pose no serious danger for children with epilepsy. Ideally, the floor should be carpeted or padded. Low-seated bicycles are the safest.

Horseback Riding

Horseback riding can be safe and fun for children whose seizures are well controlled or always preceded by an adequate warning. Those who have seizures that could cause them to fall off the horse can ride but must be closely supervised. Someone may need to walk alongside the horse.

Competitive horseback riding often involves galloping and jumping and should only be considered for children with well-controlled epilepsy.

Contact Sports

Contact sports such as football, basketball, soccer, rugby, and ice hockey are generally safe for children with epilepsy. The principal concern with contact sports is the chance of head or bodily injury, but children with epilepsy are not necessarily more likely to be hurt than other children. If an absence or complex partial seizure were to occur during a game, there is a small chance of injury if someone were to tackle the child, for instance, during the seizure. Tackle football, rugby, and ice hockey have a higher incidence of injuries than most other sports, and participation in them should be limited to children with well-controlled seizures. However, a child who has occasional or even frequent seizures can play touch football in the back yard.

Wrestling may be safe for children with well-controlled seizures or seizures that do not impair consciousness or motor control. It can be dangerous for other children with epilepsy.

Some forms of gymnastics are dangerous for children with epilepsy. Only those with well-controlled seizures should consider performing on the high bar, uneven parallel bars, balance beam, vaults, or rings. Other gymnastic events, such as floor routines and the pommel horse, pose little risk. The parallel bars are of intermediate risk; the risk reflects the specific exercises being done. Climbing a rope more than 5 feet off the ground without a harness can be dangerous if seizures are not well controlled.

23 | Education of Children with Epilepsy

M ost children with epilepsy have normal intelligence, but some do not do well academically. When this happens, it is important to find out why. Neurologic impairment, frequent seizures, or side effects of AEDs can affect school performance. If a child is doing well in school, there is no reason to worry about the effects of epilepsy on learning. If the teacher reports problems or if parents notice that performance is slipping, identify the problem. It may be an attention deficit with distractibility, excessive tiredness from medications, poor sleep, or a specific learning disability, which may or may not be related to the epilepsy (see Chapter 20). Obtain an educational assessment. Parents have the right to request an assessment of their child's problems and needs.

The Individuals with Disabilities Education Act (IDEA), discussed later, provides legal guarantees for educating children with handicaps. The child has the right to be taught in a regular classroom environment as much as possible. The child has the right to be included in social activities and other activities provided by the school. Parents have the right to be directly involved planning the child's education.

Attending Regular Classes

Most children with epilepsy attend regular classes, even though in some cases they need special aides to work with them. Regular classes offer the opportunity for children with epilepsy and other disorders to enjoy their education and to be in the social environment of children without disabilities. Mainstream classes expose the child to a wider array of opportunities, socially and academically and foster the feeling of being a kid, rather than a child with a disability. It helps emphasize the potential to learn and accomplish all the things that other children can.

Regular classes may present problems for a child with epilepsy. Children can be cruel—teasing, excluding, etc. Other parents may even forbid their children to play with a child who has epilepsy. If problems occur, ask the school to conduct an educational program so that the children can better understand epilepsy.

Special Education

Special education programs are designed to meet the needs of children with disabilities by supplementing or adapting the regular curriculum. Instruction may take place in regular classrooms or in separate facilities for all or part of the day. Students may also be assigned to special programs in physical education, occupational and physical rehabilitation, music programs, home instruction, or instruction in hospitals.

If a child is not doing well in mainstream classes, parents should meet with the teachers to identify the problems. A comprehensive evaluation (medical, educational, neuropsychological) with communication between the various parties may help identify the cause.

Schools are required to deliver services in the "least restrictive environment," meaning the regular classroom, for as much of the day as possible. Some children require many special classes or a special school, and emotional issues often arise when children are removed from the mainstream. Other special needs children may have severe emotional or behavioral problems and provide poor models. If problematic, this issue should be addressed. Parents and teachers should emphasize that the child is special, not handicapped, disabled, or less bright.

The Individuals with Disabilities Act

The IDEA ensures that all handicapped children receive appropriate education at no cost and in the least restrictive environment. All states that receive federal funds under this act must follow the rules for identifying, evaluating, and providing services to eligible children between 3 and 21 years of age. Federal funds are also provided to the states to develop early intervention services for infants and toddlers with physical or mental conditions that are likely to cause developmental delay.

This act recognizes the special needs of children with disabilities. This group includes children with epilepsy, mental retardation, hearing and visual impairments (not limited to deafness and blindness), serious emotional disorders, orthopedic impairments, autism, traumatic brain injury, learning disabilities, and other impairments. Children may qualify who have only epilepsy. To qualify for service, the disorder must adversely affect the child's educational capacity to the degree that special education or related services are required.

In some children, although their epilepsy is not disabling and their intelligence is normal, other problems may require special attention. These include impairments of attention, reading, arithmetic learning, motor skills, memory, and behavior. They are often identified at a young age, permitting early intervention and treatment.

IDEA requires that children with disabilities be educated in the "least restrictive environment." This means that a child has the right to be educated in the classroom with children who do not have disabilities, to the maximum extent that such placement meets the child's educational needs. IDEA requires that schools provide all the additional services needed to help children with disabilities benefit from special education. These services include transportation, audiology and speech therapy, psychological evaluation and treatment, physical and occupational therapy, recreation, therapeutic recreation, social work services, counseling, early identification and assessment of disabling conditions, and medical evaluations. For children with epilepsy, related services include education for teachers and school nurses about epilepsy, how to administer medications, and first aid for seizures.

IDEA states that a child with disabilities must have a written individualized educational plan (IEP) constructed jointly by the parents and school personnel. The IEP is a written report describing the child's present level of development, the short-term and annual goals of the special education program, the specific educational services the child will receive, the date services will start and their expected duration, standards for determining whether the goals of the educational program are being met, and the extent to which the child can participate in regular educational programs.

The Rehabilitation Act of 1973, Section 504

Section 504 of The Rehabilitation Act of 1973 provides education rights for children and adults with disabilities. This antidiscrimination law makes it illegal for any program or activity receiving federal funding to exclude or discriminate against qualified people with handicaps. It also requires that reasonable accommodations be made by educational institutions.

Section 504 covers "qualified" people with handicaps—not only children of school age but also persons of any other age during which state law requires that such services be provided to people with handicaps. This may include adult educational services as well as college, graduate school, and technical schools.

IV Epilepsy in Adults

24 | Mental Handicap and Cerebral Palsy

C hildren with epilepsy who also have mental handicap (a term preferred over "mental retardation") or cerebral palsy present a wide range of problems. Mental handicap refers to below average intellectual ability; these children are often impaired in their ability to understand, communicate, solve problems, and function in social settings. Cerebral palsy refers to a disorder with impaired movement, causing problems with standing or walking, weakness, coordination, and muscle spasms. Children with cerebral palsy may have normal or below average intelligence. Mental handicap and cerebral palsy can also be associated with vision, hearing, and speech problems and possibly some physical deformity or emotional disturbance. Management of children with epilepsy and mental handicap or cerebral palsy requires the combined effort of doctors, therapists, and parents.

Acceptance and Adjustment

The way in which the parents adjust to the situation is crucial for the future welfare of their handicapped child as well as the whole family. The child with mental handicap or cerebral palsy and epilepsy has the same emotional needs as other children. He or she needs love but not smothering, care but not overindulgence, and, above all, opportunities for achievement, self-control, and social growth toward an independent place in adult society.

Adjusting to the shock of being told about the child's handicap is difficult, but families can receive assistance, support, and education from United Cerebral Palsy (www.ucp.org) or The Arc of the United States (www.TheArc.org), a national organization for people with mental retardation and related developmental disabilities and their families.

Mental Handicap

Mental handicap means slowed or delayed mental development. Children with mental handicap can learn; they just learn at a slower rate than average. Approximately 2% of children in the general population have a mental handicap; approximately 25% of children with cerebral palsy and 9% of children with epilepsy have a mental handicap. For those children who have epilepsy, mental handicap is more common with the following factors: early age when seizures begin (especially before age 2 years), prolonged duration of epilepsy, multiple seizure types, and use of several AEDs in high dosages.

Intelligence tests measure a broad range of cognitive functions like math, reasoning and logic, and spatial skills, as well as the fund of knowledge. IQ tests are imperfect. Neurologic disorders can falsely depress scores. Children with epilepsy may be slowed by medication or by seizures. Those with cerebral palsy may be penalized because their movement impairments interfere with test-taking performance. Therefore, intelligence testing may not accurately indicate a child's true potential.

Mental handicap is classified as mild (IQ of 69 –55), moderate (IQ of 54–40), severe (IQ of 39–25), and profound (IQ of less than 25). If a child with epilepsy scores in the mentally handicapped range, his or her development will probably be slower than that of other children of the same age. However, children with mental handicap have a wide range of abilities.

The IQ score is one measure of intelligence. Psychologists can also measure a child's adaptive level, or ability to manage common daily activities such as feeding, dressing, toileting, and social interaction. Handicapped children with movement problems may be delayed in these areas. Obtaining an accurate picture of a child's potential requires an assessment by professionals from different fields and integrating the observations and test results.

Early intervention and special education programs can reduce the impact of mental handicap. Programs can tailor the curriculum so that children can learn at a rate that gives them confidence in their emerging new abilities. Recognizing a child's developmental strengths and weaknesses is key to planning an educational program that can achieve the child's potential. Skill development, not high scores on intelligence tests, is the goal.

Cerebral Palsy

About 30% of all children with cerebral palsy have epilepsy. A much smaller proportion of those with epilepsy have cerebral palsy. Epilepsy and cerebral palsy are separate disorders, but both can result from the same abnormality of the brain. The two conditions can co-exist, but one does not cause the other.

Cerebral palsy is a descriptive name for a group of disorders that affect control of movement and result from brain and spinal cord disease. The major problems for children with cerebral palsy are poor muscle control such as difficulty in holding up the head; delay in walking or inability to walk; incoordination; muscle tightness; and muscle spasms. Mental handicap occurs in approximately one third of children with cerebral palsy. The disorder is referred to as "stable" or "static" because it does not worsen over time. The abnormality may occur while the fetus is in the womb, around birth, or during the first year of life. Some children are not diagnosed until months or years later; symptoms vary in severity depending on the type and degree of abnormality involved.

Independence for Persons with Epilepsy and Cerebral Palsy

Children with epilepsy and cerebral palsy who have average or near average intelligence and mild physical problems usually achieve independence during later adolescence and adulthood. Children with mental and physical problems often depend on others to some extent for the rest of their lives. The parents of these children should try to help them become as independent as possible. Services can be provided through the school system, employment programs, and residential or community-based programs. In addition, programs such as the Special Olympics (www. specialolympics.org) can allow these children to participate in athletics and excel at their own level.

Education and Training

"Education" of children with cerebral palsy and epilepsy can begin shortly after birth. Many children receive services through infant stimulation programs soon after the diagnosis is made. The best infant programs almost always involve the parents as teachers of their own children. Some programs include specialists such as physical or speech therapists in addition to specially trained teachers.

Vocational Training Programs

The Individuals with Disabilities Education Act (IDEA) (see Chapter 23) makes services and training available to people with severe disabilities. They are eligible even if the most they will achieve is "supported employment," which means employment in a setting with a job coach, special training, or other services that allow an individual to perform work. The department of vocational rehabilitation in each state, sometimes called "DVR," "OVR," or "Voc Rehab," is charged with carrying out the law (see Chapter 30). Under these programs, adults with epilepsy and cerebral palsy can continue to receive vocational education after they reach age 21.

25 | Living with Epilepsy

S hould adults with epilepsy restrict their activities of daily living? If so, how much? Safety and an active life must be balanced. Decisions about driving, employment, household responsibilities, swimming, and other activities must consider the individual situation. For persons with rare or fully controlled seizures, most activities can be safely pursued. For those who have frequent seizures that impair consciousness, certain activities must be restricted.

Risk-Benefit Decisions

Risk-benefit decisions regarding activities are not unique to people with epilepsy. High-risk activities like skydiving, scuba diving, motorcycle riding, or fighting fires can potentially cause injury or death, yet millions of people participate in them every year. Those who do so feel that the benefits—enjoyment, economical transportation, employment, or helping others—outweigh the risks. Many more of us engage in lower-risk activities such as driving a car or snorkeling. Our decisions reflect our personal philosophy of life.

Seizure control heavily influences risk-benefit decisions for people with epilepsy. If seizures are well controlled, the situation is similar to someone without epilepsy. For persons with frequent, uncontrolled seizures, activities such as swimming and bike riding can be carried out with precautions, but other activities such as driving a car are unsafe and can endanger others. The most difficult decisions involve persons who have occasional seizures.

Prevention of Seizure-Related Injuries

Most seizures do not cause physical injury. Unfortunately, serious injuries can occur during tonic-clonic, tonic, or atonic seizures. During these attacks, falls can cause bruises or cuts, bone fractures, chipped teeth, sprained joints, or dislocated shoulders. People with frequent, uncontrolled seizures that cause loss of muscle control or diminished awareness of their surroundings should take special precautions in the kitchen. Also, they should not work in places where they could be injured by heat, electricity, or dangerous equipment (such as an electric saw), unless special safety features are in place or unless they *always* have a warning (aura) of an approaching seizure.

Prevention is the best strategy for avoiding seizure-related injuries. When cooking, persons with frequent seizures may be safer using a microwave oven or putting guards around an open flame. Whenever possible, they should bring individual dishes to the source of hot food rather than carrying kettles or saucepans. Other safeguards in the home include carpeting the bathroom, putting a temperature monitor on showerheads, lowering the temperature of the water heater, putting guards around radiators, using a laundry for clothes that have to be ironed, avoiding electric carving knives and slicing machines, and living in a single-story house or a first-floor or elevator-served apartment to avoid falls on stairs.

Seizure-Alert Dogs

Dogs may "sense" when a seizure is coming. The dog may alert its owner or others by whining, pawing, or in other ways. This distinctive behavior can alert and warn the person or others that a seizure may soon occur. It is possible that dogs can detect some change (for instance, an odor or tone of the voice) that warns them of an approaching seizure.

There is no scientific evidence as to whether dogs can really "sense" an impending seizure, including how often they are correct when they indicate that a seizure is coming and how often they fail to indicate an approaching seizure.

Several commercial groups train and sell seizure-alert dogs. The cost often exceeds $2000. The Delta Society (deltasociety.org) and UCB Pharma, Inc's caniue assistant program can provide helpful information.

Quality of Life

> A 40-year-old married man with two children went to an epileptologist. He had juvenile myoclonic epilepsy for more than 25 years. He was treated with high doses of two antiepileptic drugs, which caused him to sleep 12 hours a night, yet he felt constantly tired. He complained that he was "always a bit foggy, a little down and depressed." He continued to have two or three tonic-clonic seizures a year. The epileptologist took the old drugs away and prescribed another antiepileptic drug. The man is seizure-free and reports: "I am awake, my spirits are great. I can think."

The concept of "quality of life" is relatively new in medicine. It is the patient's, not the doctor's, perspectives on an illness and its effects on life. Although it would seem that the patient's and doctor's views would be similar, they can be quite different. Quality-of-life studies can offer new insights into the effect of disorders and treatments and into ways of improving patients' lives.

Quality of life is often impaired in persons with epilepsy, but doctors may not be aware of it. Some doctors consider occasional seizures "acceptable" and minor medication side effects medications "tolerable." Of course, in some cases, seizures cannot be fully controlled, and side effects invariably occur despite the doctor's best attempts to adjust the medications. Too often, however, the doctor does not aggressively try to control the seizures further or to reduce the side effects. The problem is often one of perception: The doctor does not see a problem worthy of attention, but the patient does. There is a gap in communication. A person who has occasional seizures appears "fine" but may have restrictions or problems with driving, employment, finances, social and family life, and self-esteem. Fear of another seizure may be the person's greatest disability.

Achieving the best quality of life is a challenge. Tolerating an occasional seizure may be better than daily side effects needed for full control; others prefer the cost of full control. There is no "right" answer; the key is the dialogue to find the best answer for the individual patient. Doctors must pay greater attention to patients' expectations and their actual experiences of living with epilepsy. Patients must help doctors to understand how epilepsy and its treatment affect their lives.

Motor Vehicle Driving

A driver's license is often a passport to adulthood in this country. In both rural and suburban areas, access to a motor vehicle is often essential for independence and employment. Even in many urban areas, driving is required for some jobs or recreation.

Driving is a privilege, and applicants must meet their state's criteria to qualify for a driver's license. Applicants in all states must be older than a minimum age, must not have a medical disorder that would make driving dangerous, and must pass a written test, a vision test, and a driving test.

Licensure of Persons with Epilepsy

State laws determine which medical conditions disqualify someone from obtaining a driver's license. The laws protect public safety and grant the privilege of driving to people who are the least likely to have an accident.

Absence or complex partial seizures while driving can be just as deadly as tonic-clonic seizures. The risk of injury or death can extend beyond the driver and passengers to pedestrians and people in other vehicles. The rate of motor vehicle accidents for people with epilepsy is higher than average, but much less than for alcohol intoxication. Some accidents involving epilepsy are caused by people, especially men, who drive without a license or who fail to report their epilepsy when applying for a license.

To obtain a driver's license in most states, a person with epilepsy must be free of seizures that affect consciousness and motor control for a certain period and must submit a doctor's statement of opinion that the person can drive safely. The seizure-free period varies from state to state. Although some states require a period of at least 1 year seizure-free, most consider exceptions that would permit someone to drive after a shorter interval. A conference of professional and lay epilepsy organizations recommended a seizure-free period of 3 months for driving privileges.

The Review and Decision Process

The state's department of motor vehicles reviews medical information submitted by the applicant. In complex cases, or those in which the decision is uncertain, the information is usually forwarded to a consulting doctor or medical advisory board. Most states have such a board, which may also hear appeals concerning decisions to deny or revoke driver's licenses.

Decisions made by the motor vehicle department can be appealed by requesting an administrative hearing before the medical advisory board or another designated body. If the administrative decision is not favorable, the applicant can request a review by a judge within a specified period.

In some states, someone with persistent seizures may be allowed to drive if the seizures do not impair consciousness or control of movement, occur only during sleep, are consistently preceded by an aura, are restricted to a certain time of the day (such as within an hour after awakening), or occur only when the AEDs were reduced or stopped on the advice of a doctor. A letter from the doctor confirming the presence and consistency of these features is often required. If a driver's license is revoked because of a breakthrough seizure caused by extenuating circumstances (reduction of medication on a doctor's advice or unusual stress such as the death of a loved one), the driver may appeal the decision. Evidence that the person takes the prescribed medications is often required, and the blood AED level is usually provided to show compliance.

Some states grant a restricted license to persons who do not meet the requirements for a regular driver's license. This license may allow a person with epilepsy or other disabilities to drive under certain conditions, such as during daytime only, to and from work within a certain distance from the home, or only during an emergency.

Commercial Driver's Licenses

The U.S. Department of Transportation (DOT) prohibits anyone with epilepsy from driving a truck between states. Regulations for driving a truck or bus within one state vary from state to state. Some states prohibit any person with a history of epilepsy from driving a commercial vehicle. Others are more reasonable and review each case individually.

Maintaining a Driver's License

Most states that grant driver's licenses to people with epilepsy require periodic medical reports. These reports document that seizure control remains good and that the person is taking or does not need to take medications. If the seizures have stopped or have been controlled for more than 2–5 years, most states will no longer require periodic medical reports.

If seizures recur and impair consciousness or control of movement, it is imperative to stop driving and consult the doctor, who may be able to suggest changes in lifestyle (such as more sleep) or adjustments in medications that may restore seizure control.

Potential Liability and Physician Reporting

A person with epilepsy may be civilly or criminally liable for a motor vehicle accident caused by seizures. Liability may occur when a person drives against medical advice, without a valid license, without notifying the state department of motor vehicles of the medical condition, or with the knowledge that he or she is prohibited from driving.

Six states (California, Delaware, Nevada, New Jersey, Oregon, and Pennsylvania) have "mandatory reporting laws," requiring that doctors report persons with epilepsy and other disorders that may make driving hazardous. Doctors may be liable for negligence if they fail to report a person with epilepsy who is later involved in a motor vehicle accident. In states without such laws, however, the question of whether a doctor should report a patient who may be driving unsafely presents a difficult conflict between public safety and the confidentiality of the doctor–patient relationship.

The specifics of when a doctor must report someone can be vague, however. In New Jersey, for example, the law states that the doctor will report any person 16 years of age or older for recurrent convulsive seizures *or* for recurrent periods of unconsciousness *or* for impairment or loss of motor coordination due to conditions such as, but not limited to, epilepsy in any of its forms when such conditions persist or recur despite medical treatments. This law is open to some interpretation—for example, exactly what constitutes "medical treatments." The plural usage indicates that more than one treatment has failed to control the seizures but does not specify how many dosage adjustments or medications must have been tried.

Mandatory reporting laws should be repealed, as was done by Connecticut in 1990. However, if a physician in Connecticut cares for a person whose seizures are so poorly controlled that driving would present a serious risk to public safety and the person continues to drive, the doctor can report the person with immunity from lawsuit by the patient. Mandatory reporting can destroy the doctor–patient relationship. In many cases, those who believe that they "must" drive lie to the doctor about their condition to keep their license. This creates the worst of both worlds: the person is not receiving the best medical care and is driving. The doctor and patient should work together.

Sports and Other Physical Activities

Persons with well-controlled seizures, seizures occurring only during sleep, or seizures that are always preceded by a warning should have few or no restrictions on physical activities. For persons who continue to have complex partial or tonic-clonic seizures, even if they are preceded by warnings, some restrictions should apply, such as skydiving or deep scuba dives. People whose seizures are not fully controlled can pursue most sporting activities, including water skiing, sailing, wind-surfing, snorkeling, bicycling, gymnastics, soccer, football, baseball, handball, squash, tennis, basketball, volleyball, archery, skiing, sledding, hiking, and many others. When a person is engaged in any of these activities, certain precautions can help to minimize the risk of injury. For example, a life vest reduces the risk of drowning during water sports. Having someone nearby who is familiar with the condition and with basic lifesaving skills is often wise. Snorkeling can also be enjoyed by persons with seizures, but they must use caution about where they snorkel. Although diving from the edge of a pool, dock, or low diving board is generally safe, diving off a high diving board can be dangerous.

Hiking can be safely pursued by persons with recurrent seizures, but mountain climbing can be dangerous. Whether a person uses ropes or climbs along difficult paths, the activity can be dangerous even for the most alert and agile climber. A brief lapse of concentration or a small problem with control of movement could be deadly. Climbers should carefully consider the specific trail or mountain.

Hunting can be safely pursued by persons with epilepsy. When hunting, someone should stay close by a person whose seizures are not fully controlled. If the person has a warning of a seizure, he or she should lay the gun down immediately. If a warning does not always occur, it may be best only to load the rifle shortly before shooting, and then to unload it if no shot is taken.

Smoking

Smoking tobacco is not known to have any definite effects on seizure control. But persons with epilepsy not only are susceptible to all the usual effects of smoking but also are at increased risk of injury or death from fire.

Consider what happened to one of my patients and her daughter. A 35-year-old woman with absence and tonic-clonic seizures lived with her 5-year-old daughter. One evening, the woman had a tonic-clonic seizure while smoking. When she awoke in the hospital, she had first-degree burns on a large part of her arms and body. Her daughter suffered severe smoke inhalation, is severely retarded, and unable to walk. The woman stopped smoking and went through a long emotional recovery.

Romantic Relationships and Marriage

Persons with well-controlled or infrequent seizures should have no serious problems dating or developing and maintaining a stable, intimate relationship. Uncontrolled seizures make dating and romantic relationships difficult, but success is very possible. All persons with epilepsy face some important questions: Do I tell this person that I have epilepsy? When should I tell him or her? How much should I tell?

There is no reason to rush the disclosure of epilepsy. Unless the seizures are so frequent that one might occur on the first date, wait until the ice is broken and trust and openness have developed. Try to tell the other person face to face. The way in which the disorder is presented is often how the other person will see it. Be honest and talk about how you have been affected. Allow the other person to react to what he or she has heard. Epilepsy should not be the sole focus of the conversation. Discuss it and then move on to other subjects. Like everyone else, a person with epilepsy is defined by many traits and attributes; epilepsy should not become the defining feature.

Anyone who dates and gets involved in romantic relationships will experience rejection. Some prospective partners may say no to the first date or the second date, and others may break up the relationship after an extended period. People are rejected because of physical characteristics, personality traits, social beliefs, and other reasons. Epilepsy may contribute to the reasons for rejection by some people, but it may be "attractive" to others who have a need to nurture or care for someone.

Sex Life

Persons with epilepsy can enjoy all the sexual feelings and pleasures others enjoy. Most persons with epilepsy have normal sex lives. There is no convincing evidence that seizures are more likely to occur during sexual activities. Rarely, seizures may be more likely to occur during or shortly after physical exertion and intense emotional experiences.

Sexual dysfunction, a common problem in the general population, refers to an inability to experience sexual feelings and arousal or to perform sexual activities. These problems include decreased libido, or a lower level of interest in sexual activity, as well as the failure of a man to achieve an erection (impotence) or the inability of a man or woman to achieve an orgasm (anorgasmia). Women with epilepsy are more likely than other women to experience painful intercourse and sexual dissatisfaction. Some people with epilepsy with reduced libido do not consider it a problem. More often, a spouse feels that the partner's interest in sex is less than normal.

The AEDs that induce liver enzymes can cause or aggravate sexual dysfunction. These drugs include carbamazepine, phenobarbital, phenytoin, and primidone; oxcarbazepine and topiramate can also induce the liver enzymes and may contribute to these problems. The enzyme-inducing

AEDs increase the liver's metabolism of testosterone, leading to lower testosterone levels, which are strongly linked with sexual dysfunction (decreased interest and impotence) in men. The effect of these AEDs on women's sexual function has not been adequately studied.

Other factors can contribute to sexual dysfunction: underlying brain disorder (such as head trauma), the chronic effects of seizures, and psychological factors. Sexual dysfunction is more common in patients with poorly controlled epilepsy. Approximately 20% of men with epilepsy who do not take enzyme-inducing AEDs report impaired sexual function. Depression and drugs used to treat depression can impair sexual function. For example, the selective serotonin reuptake inhibitors (SSRIs) (e.g., Zoloft [sertaline], paroxetine [Paxil], and Prozac [fluoxetine]) can impair sexual function in 30–60% of patients. Although this side effect may resolve within 4–6 weeks, if it persists, reducing the dose of the SSRI, altering the timing of the daily dose or a 2–day drug holiday (for sertaline and paroxetine) may be helpful. Other antidepressant agents should be considered: bupropion (Wellbutrin) and nefazodone (Serzone) cause sexual dysfunction in 10% or less of patients. However, bupropion may promote seizures, especially at doses of over 300 mg/day.

If sexual dysfunction is a problem, a person should discuss it with the doctor, and referral to a gynecologist, urologist, sex therapists, or other specialist may be helpful. Counseling should always be considered, especially if psychological or marital issues are suspected. Drugs used to treat erectile dysfunction (impotence)—Viagra (sildenafil) and Cialis (tadalafil)—appear to be safe for epilepsy patients and do not interact with AEDs.

Adolescent girls and women with epilepsy should be aware that AEDs can cause birth defects (see Chapter 26). They also need to be educated about the different types of birth control and the interaction between AEDs and birth control pills (see Chapter 12). Adolescent girls with epilepsy have a higher frequency of unplanned pregnancy than females their age in the general population.

Fertility

Most men and women with epilepsy have normal sex lives, are fertile, and have perfectly healthy children. Nevertheless, epilepsy, its treatment, and associated disorders may affect fertility and reproduction. Men and women with epilepsy have fewer children than people in the general population. Men with epilepsy may have slightly reduced fertility. Hormonal changes associated with the seizures may contribute. In addition, sperm production may be reduced in men who take some AEDs. Women with epilepsy also have higher rates of infertility than women in the general population. The effects of AEDs, tonic-clonic seizures, and irregular menstrual cycles probably contribute.

The polycystic ovary syndrome is characterized by high levels of testosterone in the blood, increased hair growth (hirsutism), multiple ovarian cysts, irregular menstruation, and lack of ovulation. Many of the affected women are obese. This syndrome is more common among women with epilepsy. Valproic acid can cause this syndrome in some women.

Infertile couples in which one member, or both, have epilepsy should consult with an infertility specialist. Common causes of infertility, such as endometriosis (abnormal location of the lining of the womb) in women or a varicocele (abnormal collection of veins in the scrotal sac) in men, should be investigated and treated. Infertility should never be dismissed as simply a problem of epilepsy or AEDs.

26 | Contraception, Pregnancy, and Menopause

The Childbearing Years

Women with epilepsy face special challenges: effects of the menstrual cycle on seizures (see Chapter 7), interactions of AEDs and hormone contraception, concerns about effects of epilepsy or AEDs on their pregnancy and unborn child, and changes with menopause. Although it is best to avoid medications during pregnancy, most women with epilepsy are unable to safely stop their AEDs during pregnancy. Table 26.1 highlights three important principles for all women with epilepsy regarding pregnancy.

Contraception

Contraceptives methods include barrier, hormonal therapies, and intrauterine devices. Barrier methods, including condoms and diaphragm caps, are not affected by AEDs (Table 26.2). Similarly, intrauterine devices (IUDs) and intrauterine systems (IUSs; an intrauterine device that releases progesterone directly into the womb) are not affected by AEDs. Hormonal contraceptives include the standard combination birth control pill (estrogen and progesterone), the mini-pill (progesterone only), progesterone injections (Depo-Provera), progesterone implants (Implanon), or patch (estrogen and progestin [a form of progesterone]). The effectiveness of these hormonal

Table 26.1. Pregnancy for Women with Epilepsy (WWE): Basic Principles

1. The large majority of WWE have healthy pregnancies and babies, although they are at increased risk.

2. All WWE of childbearing potential should discuss pregnancy issues with her physician prior to pregnancy.

3. Don't stop or reduce antiepileptic drug(s) without talking with your physician.

Table 26.2. Interaction of AEDs and Contraception

Drugs that may reduce the effectiveness of hormonal contraception	Drugs that do not reduce the effectiveness of hormonal contraception
Carbamazepine	Benzodiazepines
Oxcarbazepine*	Gabapentin
Phenobarbital	Lamotrigine**
Phenytoin	Levetiracetam
Primidone	Pregabalin
Topiramate*	Tiagabine
	Valproic acid
	Vigabatrin
	Zonisamide

* Effects of oxcarbazepine and topiramate on hormonal contraceptives occur at higher dosages.

** Lamotrigine levels can be reduced by hormones.

contraceptives may be reduced by enzyme-inducing AEDs, thus making pregnancy more likely. The interaction of enzyme-inducing AEDs and the estrogen and progesterone levels released by vaginal rings (NuvaRing) over a 21-day period is uncertain; until better data are available, these should not be considered reliable for women on these medications. The morning after pill is a very concentrated form of the birth control pill (levonorgestrel). If a woman is taking an enzyme-inducing AED, she should take one pill immediately and another one 12 hours later.

Planning Before Pregnancy

Planning for pregnancy is not limited to women who are actively intending to become pregnant, but should include all women of childbearing age.

Many babies are born each year to women with epilepsy who were not planning on becoming pregnant.

Defining the potential dangers and ways of reducing risks is a starting point for family planning. The risks associated with pregnancy for women with epilepsy are fairly well defined. Many of the steps to reduce the problems for both the mother and the child must be taken before the pregnancy begins. There should be good communication among the couple, the neurologist, and the obstetrician to maximize seizure control and the chances for a healthy pregnancy and baby. More than 90% of women with epilepsy have healthy babies.

Risk of Epilepsy in the Baby

Children whose parents have epilepsy have a slightly higher risk of developing epilepsy. The lifetime risk of developing epilepsy in the general population is approximately 3%. If the father has epilepsy and the mother does not, the risk to the children is only slightly higher than 3%. If the mother has epilepsy and the father does not, the risk is higher but still under 5%. The highest risk is in women with primary generalized epilepsy. If both parents have epilepsy, the risk is a bit higher than if only one parent has the condition.

A couple in which one or even both partners have epilepsy should not decide to forgo having children because of fear that the children will have epilepsy. The risk of epilepsy is low; many children outgrow epilepsy, and the seizures are usually controlled with a single drug.

Birth Defects and Antiepileptic Drugs

The healthiest women have a 1.5–2.5% chance of having a baby with a major birth defect. The chance increases to 3–6% in women with epilepsy taking most AEDs as monotherapy (a single AED). The major cause of the increased risk appears to be the AED, but genetic factors may contribute. A few studies suggest that certain birth defects are slightly more common among children of parents who have epilepsy, even if the parents did not take AEDs.

Antiepileptic drugs taken by the mother shortly before conception and during the first 3 months of pregnancy pose the greatest danger of producing congenital birth defects in the developing baby. Women with epilepsy are faced with a difficult decision. AEDs during pregnancy pose risks for the baby, but most women need to continue taking them. It is an understandable but potentially dangerous practice to reduce or stop medication without a doctor's recommendation. Seizures can be dangerous to both the mother and the baby—and to others if the woman drives.

The first trimester (3 months) of pregnancy, especially days 21–56, is the critical period for the development of the baby's major organ systems. The second and third trimesters (the last 6 months) are important for growth and maturation. In a small percentage of fetuses, AED exposure during the first trimester can cause major birth defects such as cleft lip and cleft palate (a gap in the middle of the lip or palate) and structural defects of the heart, brain, spinal cord, gastrointestinal system, reproductive system, urinary system, and the skeletal system. These defects are serious, but often the child can live normally after surgery or other treatments. Minor malformations may also result from AED exposure. These include widely spaced eyes, a small and upturned nose, and short fingers and toes. Minor defects are not rare in the general population and may disappear after the first year of life.

The new AEDs (felbamate, gabapentin, lamotrigine, levetiracetam, oxcarbazepine, tiagabine, topiramate, and zonisamide) are now being studied in pregnant women. More safety information will hopefully come from several registries for women taking AEDs during pregnancy. Pregnant women who are taking AEDs are encouraged to contact the North American (888-233-2334, or *www.aedpregnancyregistry.org*) or other international registries and provide information that may help define the safety of their future pregnancies, as well as the pregnancies of other women. Communication with the registry is confidential.

Information from the various pregnancy registries indicates some similarities but also differences. Polytherapy is consistently more dangerous to the fetus than monotherapy. Valproic acid has uniformly come out as the AED associated with the highest risk of major birth defects and developmental delays in children exposed during their mother's pregnancy. The data for lamotrigine are conflicting; several studies have found little to no risk, while one found increasing risk with increasing dose (especially over 300 mg/day) but other studies have not seen a dose effect. Another study found an increased risk for cleft lip/palate, but this has not been confirmed by other registries. Available data suggest that levetiracetam monotherapy may be safe, but more data is needed.

Treatment with one AED in the lowest dosage that will control the seizures presents the least risk for the baby's development. Any woman of childbearing age taking two or more AEDs and who would consider having a baby if she became pregnant should ask her doctor if she could be treated with one medication. More than one drug may be necessary for seizure control, but many can be safely treated with one drug, and some can remain seizure-free with lower dosages than usually taken. Women who are thinking of discontinuing or reducing the dose of their AEDs may find no better time to try, under a doctor's supervision, than before pregnancy.

Knowing the approximate risks is not always reassuring. Some couples are relieved to learn that the risk of major birth defects is small. But others focus on the relative percentages, noting that the risk of birth defects is approximately double that of the general population, even though the percentages are still small. Most experts recommend that women and men with epilepsy should have children if they want. However, those with uncontrolled seizures or taking high doses of several AEDs should carefully consider the risks.

Taking Vitamins

Taking vitamins before and during pregnancy may help reduce the risks of malformations in the baby. Folate (folic acid) appears to be the most important vitamin, but the best dose remains unknown. The recommended daily minimum in the general adult population is 0.4 mg, the amount found in most high-potency vitamins. For women taking AEDs, a supplemental dose of 1.0–2 mg/day is reasonable. A dose of 2–4 mg/day is reasonable for those with a history of birth defects in their family, in a previous pregnancy, or who take valproic acid. In addition to folate, women with epilepsy who may become pregnant should probably take a high-potency multivitamin pill. Some evidence links very high doses of vitamin A or D with birth defects, but the doses in a standard high-potency multivitamin should be safe.

Care During Pregnancy

Regular medical care is essential for all pregnant women. The doctor can identify common problems of pregnancy before they become serious. Because of the risk of complications during pregnancy and the potential for problems with seizure control, regular visits to both the obstetrician and the neurologist are crucial.

Excessive vaginal bleeding during pregnancy is the most common obstetrical problem in women with epilepsy. Other potential problems include abnormalities of the placenta (the organ that nourishes the baby) and complications around the time of birth, such as high blood pressure (preeclampsia) and premature delivery. Some studies, but not all, have found that the infants of women with epilepsy had more problems after birth (including a higher rate of death). However, with modern care, adverse outcomes of this kind are becoming less likely.

Taking Vitamins

In addition to a multivitamin and folate supplementation, women who are taking enzyme-inducing AEDs (for example, carbamazepine, phenobarbital, phenytoin, primidone, topiramate) should take 10–20 mg/day of vitamin K by mouth during the last 4 weeks of pregnancy. This can help prevent the possibility of internal bleeding in the newborn. Although intramuscular vitamin K is given to most babies at delivery, use of oral vitamin K by the mother is still recommended.

Effects of Pregnancy on Seizure Control

Pregnancy brings about dramatic changes in the body. It affects metabolism, fluid balance, hormone levels, and other physical functions and has a psychological impact. These changes can make seizure control unpredictable. Of women with epilepsy who become pregnant, one fifth have an increase in seizure frequency, one sixth have a reduction, and more than half have no change. Seizure activity or freedom during one pregnancy does not necessarily predict what will happen during subsequent pregnancies. Women need to take their medications as prescribed. If nausea and vomiting become a problem, the doctor should be informed immediately, because the absorption of AEDs can be seriously affected.

Drug dosages must be adjusted during pregnancy for many women with epilepsy. Monitoring blood levels of the drugs is helpful, especially for drugs such as lamotrigine and oxcarbazepine, but the patient's condi-tion is also an important guide for maintaining or changing therapy. If seizures were well controlled before pregnancy, many doctors do not increase the dosage of AEDs during the first 3 months, even if the AED blood levels decline slightly. If the frequency of seizures increases or there is a moderate to large decline in the levels, however, a higher dosage is usually needed.

The AED blood levels usually decline during pregnancy, even if the drugs are taken as prescribed. Causes for declining blood levels include decreased protein binding, increased metabolism, and increased blood volume and weight gain. The total amount of drug in the blood consists of two parts: *bound*, or attached, to proteins; and *unbound*, or floating freely. Only the unbound, or free, drug crosses from the blood to the brain and helps to control seizures. When a blood level is monitored, the results are usually the total drug level. Although the total blood levels of all AEDs are moderately reduced during pregnancy, the free levels of many drugs (phenobarbital is an exception) are usually reduced by a smaller percentage. A doctor who considered only the total drug level might predict that seizure control would worsen; the free level is a more reliable guide. The increased levels of hormones during pregnancy cause a marked reduction in lamotrigine levels, which can increase the seizure frequency. For women on lamotrigine, blood levels should be obtained every month and the dosage usually needs to be increased throughout pregnancy, often by as much as threefold, to maintain stable blood levels. The dosage needs to be readjusted after delivery as the hormone levels decline and lamotrigine levels increase.

Effects of a Woman's Seizures on the Baby

Absence seizures, simple partial seizures, or complex partial seizures during pregnancy pose no danger to the baby unless the woman injures herself during the seizure, which is rare. Convulsive (tonic-clonic) seizures in the woman, however, can occasionally be dangerous for the developing baby. However, only rare cases are documented in which a convulsive seizure harmed a baby by causing a sustained and dangerous depression in the baby's heart rate. Most women who have one or two tonic-clonic seizures during pregnancy have healthy babies. Theoretically, tonic-clonic seizures may be most dangerous to the fetus during the last trimester, when the brain is larger and needs more oxygen. Repetitive or prolonged tonic-clonic seizures (convulsive status epilepticus) can impair the supply of oxygen to the baby's brain. In a study of nearly 2000 pregnancies in women with epilepsy, there were 12 cases of convulsive status epilepticus, one of which was complicated by a stillbirth. However, the potential neurodevelopmental effects on the surviving 11 babies was not studied.

Labor and Delivery

Women with epilepsy have induced labors and cesarean deliveries ("C sections") much more often than women without epilepsy. This difference partly reflects the perceived risks of complications of labor and delivery rather than the actual risks. Women taking high dosages of AEDs may have slightly weaker contractions of the womb (uterus) during delivery, although this is unproven. Epilepsy itself is not a reason to induce labor, as most women with epilepsy can have normal, spontaneous labor and deliveries. In selected situations, however, it may be prudent to induce labor. The potential benefits of an induced labor must be weighed against the risks, which include prolonged labor as well as uterine and physical exhaustion, which can lead to the need for a cesarean section.

For women who have only simple or complex partial seizures, myoclonic seizures, or absence seizures, there should be no problems with a natural vaginal delivery. Similarly, well-controlled or infrequent tonic-clonic seizures present no reason not to try a natural vaginal delivery. However, for women who have uncontrolled tonic-clonic seizures during pregnancy or those with tonic-clonic seizures during prior labor and delivery, cesarean section may be indicated.

The frequency of seizures increases slightly during labor and delivery and the first 2 days after delivery. One to 2% of women may have tonic-clonic seizures during this period. This increase may result from the stress of labor leading to missed AED doses, sleep deprivation, hyperventilation, pain, and other medications such as meperidine (Demerol). Women should prepare for labor with a reminder to take medications as scheduled, and they should tell the doctor if they are unable to take them because of nausea or pain. Fortunately, despite many of these problems, 98% of women do not have tonic-clonic seizures around the time of delivery.

Spinal anesthesia is safe for women with epilepsy. If general anesthesia is required, it also can be given, although long-term safety for the fetus has not been established. The anesthesiologist should be informed about the woman's history of epilepsy and the AEDs she is taking.

Cognitive Development in Children of Mothers with Epilepsy

Do children of women with epilepsy have higher rates of cognitive problems? If they do, are the problems associated with genetic or nutritional factors, specific drugs, certain seizure types, or other factors? Current knowledge does not provide clear answers. Several, but not all studies suggest that children of women with epilepsy have higher rates of cognitive disorders. Some data suggest that the risk of AED effects on a child's cognition are due primarily to third trimester exposure. Four studies found that valproate was associated with higher rates of developmental delays (such as learning disorders, autism and mental handicap) in babies who were exposed during pregnancy. A recent prospective study found that the average IQ of 2-year-olds exposed to valproate was lower than those exposed to other AEDs. In several studies, carbamazepine and lamotrigine were not associated with negative cognitive effects.

The lowest effective dose of a single drug and controlling seizures during pregnancy may help minimize any potential risks.

Menopause

Menopause, which usually occurs between ages 44 and 56 years, is marked by a decline ovarian function leading to reduced estrogen and progesterone production and the end of menstrual cycles. Common symptoms during the transition into menopause include hot flashes and mood changes. The effects of menopause on seizure frequency and intensity have not been extensively studied. For most women, seizure activity does not significantly change, although it can worsen or improve. Care around the time of menopause for women with epilepsy should be individualized.

The benefits and risks of hormone replacement therapy (HRT) during and after menopause are complex. Estrogen replacement can reduce hot flashes and prevent cardiovascular disease and osteoporosis. Estrogen replacement can also increase the risk of uterine and breast cancer, leading many experts to caution against or limit HRT use. HRT with the commonly used Prempro caused a dose-related increase in seizure activity in one study.

Androgens (male sex hormones) such as testosterone are occasionally used to improve libido (sexual desire), emotional well-being, and bone density in postmenopausal women. However, androgen supplementation after menopause may have adverse effects and is not recommended routinely. Long-term follow-up studies are limited.

27 | Parenting by People with Epilepsy

F ew other joys equal those of parenthood, and epilepsy should not prevent someone from becoming a parent.

Caring for Infants and Children

Caring for a baby or child means loss of freedom and personal time, as well as responsibility. Persons with well-controlled epilepsy have no restrictions on child care, but those with seizures that impair consciousness or control of movement must take special precautions when caring for a baby or a young child. The precautions depend on the child's age, its nature, and other circumstances.

Ideally, a parent with uncontrolled seizures should not bathe the baby alone. The baby should be placed in a safely designed baby bath and transferred to and from the bath relatively close to the floor. If the baby bath is placed inside a larger tub, the drain should be open. The bathroom should be carpeted if possible. The parent should always heed a warning of a seizure while bathing the baby.

A parent with uncontrolled seizures should be extremely careful when carrying the baby. Some get enough warning of a seizure to place the baby down safely. Others have no warning, and must be especially careful. Breast feeding and diaper changing by women who are at risk of having a seizure are best done on the floor or on a low, soft surface where the baby would be safe from falling.

The baby or young child of a parent who has epilepsy should sleep in its own crib or bed. There is a chance the child could be injured if the parent had a seizure, especially a tonic-clonic seizure, while sleeping.

As the baby becomes a toddler, other potential dangers confront a parent whose seizures are not fully controlled. For example, walking or playing near a busy street with an impulsive, active 2-year-old could be dangerous if the parent had a complex partial seizure. During the minute or two of impaired consciousness, the child might run after a ball that bounced onto the street. Although events such as this are rare, consider ways of reducing the risk. In this case, the child might be given another toy that is less likely to bounce into the street, or the child's and the parent's hands might be linked by a colorful plastic coil.

If a parent's seizures are not fully controlled, the disorder should be discussed with older children. Children understand more than adults give them credit for, and they may be aware of the seizures and frightened by them. Explaining to the children what a seizure is, why the parent takes medication, and why the children should not worry is comforting to them. As the children get older, they should be told more about epilepsy and what to do if first aid is needed.

For new parents, some sleep deprivation and stress are unavoidable, and dramatic changes in the daily schedule can easily lead to missed medications. It is important to recognize these potential problems and plan to reduce their impact. For example, a mother with epilepsy who chooses to breastfeed might use a formula supplement at night so her husband feeds the baby and she can sleep.

Breastfeeding

Breastfeeding is recommended for most women with epilepsy, because breast milk confers benefits to the baby, including protection against infection. However, the benefits of breast-feeding must be weighed against the risks when the mother takes AEDs.

Table 27.1 shows the approximate percentages of the mother's blood drug level found in breast milk. The amount of drug found in breast

Table 27.1. AEDs and Breastfeeding

Antiepileptic drug	Breast milk:maternal blood concentration (approx %)	Half-life in newborn baby (hr)
Carbamazepine	50	10–25
Ethosuximide	85	30–40
Gabapentin	160	15
Lamotrigine	60	20–25
Levetiracetam	100	15–20
Phenobarbital	50	50–350
Phenytoin	30	20–40
Primidone	80	20–50
Valproic acid	5–10	40–50
Zonisamide	50–80	70–100

milk is related to the proportion of the drug that is not bound to proteins. The more a drug is bound to proteins in the blood, the lower the amount that is free and the lower the amount found in breast milk (Table 27-1).

Phenobarbital and primidone, both barbiturates, cause the most problems with breast feeding. The baby's digestive system is good at absorbing these drugs, and they linger for an unusually long time in the baby's blood. A single dose of pheno-barbital may last more than 15 days. Because of the high amount of ethosuximide, gabapentin, and levetiracetam found in breast milk, and the active transport of gabapentin and levetiracetam into breast milk, these may also cause problems. However, for levetiracetam, blood levels in the baby are very low, likely due to rapid elimination. In breastfed babies, AEDs may cause fussy feeding habits, tiredness, and irritability. Some irritability and gas pains are normal, however, and should not be interpreted as medication effects. The mother should contact the pediatrician if she has any doubts.

If a woman takes two or more AEDs, the baby should be watched closely for signs of toxicity. The baby of a woman taking phenobarbital who breastfeeds and then stops should be observed for signs of drug withdrawal such as increased irritability, insomnia, or sweating. If these signs are observed, the pediatrician should be contacted.

28 | Employment and Military Service for People with Epilepsy

A productive and satisfying work life is important to a person's quality of life and self-esteem. Most people with epilepsy are capable of productive and gratifying employment, but they may face discrimination in the job market: stigma associated with epilepsy, misconceptions about its medical and social aspects, unfounded fears of legal and medical liability, and the misconception that people with epilepsy are not as productive as others. These biases have led to discrimination, but new laws have improved employment opportunities for people with epilepsy and other disabilities.

Protection Against Job Discrimination

The Americans with Disabilities Act (ADA) makes discrimination based on disability illegal in employment, activities of state and local governments, public and private transportation, public accommodations, and telecommunications. In the 2000 census, 20% of Americans were disabled in some way. Epilepsy is a disability, but not all people with epilepsy are protected by the ADA. The act is applicable if epilepsy substantially limits one or more major life activities (for example, caring for oneself, sleeping, working, or reproduction). If the disorder is fully controlled by medication, it is not considered a disability unless there are associated disorders or significant side effects of medication.

For people with epilepsy, several issues can rise to the "substantial level" and qualify for inclusion within the ADA:

- Seizures; not only in terms of absolute severity and frequency, but also the uncertainty and unpredictability of when seizures will occur

- Medication side effects (tiredness, dizziness, irritability, impaired attention)

- Balance between seizure control and side effects; many patients may have either an occasional breakthrough seizure or intermittent side effects. While neither alone might qualify, the combination can be a substantial disability

- Inability to drive or safely use other forms of transportation

- Lower rates of marriage and reproduction

- High rates of unemployment (25%; near 50% among those with uncontrolled seizures)

The courts often take a conservative approach to such claims. Further, the Supreme Court ruled that states cannot be forced to make accommodations for their disabled employees, since it might cost taxpayers money.

Title I of the ADA provides that people with disabilities cannot be excluded from employment unless they are unable to perform the essential requirements of the job. An employer may *not* discriminate in:

- Recruitment, advertising, and job application procedures

- Hiring, upgrading, promotion, demotion, tenure, transfer, layoff, termination, return from layoff, and rehiring

- Rates of pay or other compensation and changes in compensation

- Job assignment, job classification, position descriptions, lines of progression, structures, and seniority lists

- Leaves of absence, sick leave, or other leave

- Fringe benefits, whether or not administered by the employer

- Selection and financial support for training, including apprenticeships, professional meetings, conferences and other related activities, and selection for leaves of absence to pursue training

- Activities sponsored by the employer, including social and recreational programs

- Any other term, condition, or privilege of employment

The ADA applies to all employers, employment agencies, and labor organizations with 15 or more employees who work for each working day in each of 20 or more calendar weeks. The ADA excludes the federal government or other employers that receive a certain level of federal support (because they are subject to other similar regulations), as well as Indian tribes and private-membership clubs that are tax exempt.

In the following sections, the use of the term "employers" refers only to employers covered by the ADA. However, state and local laws can provide protection equal to or better than the ADA and cover a wider range of employers.

Criteria for Employment

Persons with epilepsy or other disabilities must be both qualified and able to perform the *essential* job functions, possibly with some change in the work environment or procedures (that is, a "reasonable accommodation"). The ADA does not require employers to change the fundamental duties of jobs to meet the needs of individuals with disabilities.

Discrimination and Segregation

Throughout history, job applicants with epilepsy have often experienced discrimination because of the stigma attached to their disorder. Current laws, however, forbid employers from disciminating against people with disabilities because of fears and myths. For example, a department store could not deny the position of salesclerk to a person with epilepsy because "we are afraid that seizures will frighten off the customers." Employees cannot be segregated because of their disability. For example, it would be illegal for a company to deny use of an employees' exercise room to an employee with epilepsy, although it may be reasonable for the company to obtain medical clearance from the employee's doctor.

Contractual Arrangements

The ADA requires employers to provide equal benefits and privileges to all employees regardless of disability. Even indirect discrimination through an outside contractual arrangement is illegal. For example, if a company signs a contract allowing its employees to use a certain health club but that club excludes people with epilepsy, the employer is violating the ADA.

Reasonable Accommodations

The ADA requires that covered employers make reasonable accommodations for people with disabilities unless the employer can show that the individual poses a direct threat to the health and safety of others or that the accommodation would impose an "undue burden" on the employer. Reasonable accommodation is defined as "any change in the work environment or in the way things are customarily done that enables an individual with a disability to enjoy equal employment opportunities." It is illegal for an employer to hire an individual who does not have a disability over an equally qualified disabled individual simply to avoid having to make a reasonable accommodation for the disabled person.

There are three categories of reasonable accommodations. These provide accommodations for (1) equal opportunity in the application process, (2) performing essential functions of the position held or desired, and (3) enjoying equal benefits and privileges of employment as are enjoyed by employees without disabilities.

A broad range of reasonable accommodations could apply to people with epilepsy. The following are some examples:

- Providing extended time to take an entrance examination

- Job restructuring; that is, redistributing *nonessential* or marginal job functions, such as driving, to other employees

- Temporary changes in job responsibilities or time required to perform certain tasks while someone is adjusting to new medications or to changes in an existing drug regimen

- Replacing a flickering light or loud banging noise if it could provoke a seizure

- Installing a safety shield around a piece of equipment

- Installing carpet on a concrete floor

- Asking a supervisor for written, as opposed to oral, instructions for someone with memory loss caused by antiepileptic medications

- Allowing an employee who experiences fatigue as an adverse effect of medications to take more frequent breaks

- Allowing an employee to take an extended break after a seizure

Determining what accommodation is reasonable can be difficult. The applicant or employee should notify the employer of his or her need for accommodation. The employer may require that the need for the accommodation be documented by a doctor's letter. The employer and the qualified person with a disability are required to undertake a "flexible, interactive process" in determining what accommodation is reasonable.

Information can be obtained from the protection and advocacy staff of the state human rights commission, the Equal Employment Opportunities Commission (EEOC), or a social worker who specializes in employment issues. Other resources for information on employment issues are the Epilepsy Foundation (EF) (800-EFA-1000), their state vocational rehabilitation agency (for the one nearest you, call 800-222-JOBS), or the Job Accommodation Network (800-526-7234 Voice/TDD).

Employee Benefits

The ADA does not require an employer to offer health benefits or other forms of insurance. But employers who do offer benefits to employees may not exclude people with disabilities and must offer the same plans or policies to all individuals. Employers may not refuse to hire persons or family members with disabilities because of a feared or actual increase in insurance costs.

Bringing a Claim of Discrimination

A person who believes that he or she has been discriminated against in the workplace should file a complaint with the EEOC (employment claim) or the Department of Justice (claims regarding public access and government services). These government agencies will then investigate and if the facts support the person's claim, they issue a "right to sue" letter.

For a claim of discrimination to be valid, the individual with a disability must establish that (1) the disability is covered under the ADA, (2) the employer in question is covered by the law, (3) the individual is qualified to perform the essential functions of the job, and (4) the employer violated one or more of the prohibitions of the act.

The employer has the burden of proof to show a valid defense to the employee's claim of discrimination. Various defenses can be used by the employer, including these two:

1. *Direct threat:* The employer must show that the applicant or employee with a disability presents "a significant risk of substantial harm to the health or safety of the individual or others that cannot be eliminated or reduced by reasonable accommodation."
2. *Undue hardship:* The employer must show that an accommodation required for the employee or applicant to do the job would be "unduly costly, extensive, substantial or disruptive, or would fundamentally alter the nature or operation of the business."

The Application Process

The ADA makes it illegal for an employer to use any job application that requires individuals to disclose their disability. Applications cannot list medical, neurological, or psychiatric disorders such as diabetes, epilepsy, or depression and ask people to check off those that apply to them. Further, a question such as, "Do you have a health condition that would affect your ability to do the job?" is also prohibited by the ADA because it is overly broad. Similarly, application forms cannot ask if someone has previously filed a workers' compensation claim. An application can ask questions about the applicant's ability to perform essential job duties.

Applicants with epilepsy may choose not to disclose that they have the disorder if it is under good control. However, seizures that interfere with consciousness or control of movement are potentially dangerous if the person drives, works with dangerous equipment or in a dangerous setting, or has a position (such as a ski lift operator or lifeguard) with responsibility for the safety of others. The doctor is often asked to write a letter regarding the safety of the person with epilepsy in a specific situation. Unfortunately, no one can guarantee safety.

The Job Interview

The ADA prohibits employers from asking any interview question that would require individuals to reveal their disability. The employer may ask about the applicant's ability to perform both essential and marginal job-related functions, but these questions cannot be phrased in terms of disability. For example, a flower shop owner who needs a delivery person can ask whether the applicant has a driver's license, which is essential for the job. If the response is no, the employer cannot ask if the applicant has epilepsy or a visual impairment. The employer cannot refuse to hire someone with a disability because he or she cannot perform marginal or nonessential job functions.

During the interview, the employer may ask if an accommodation will be needed during the application process. If the applicant tells the employer that he or she has epilepsy and that the medications affect the ability to respond quickly to written questions, then the employer may ask how much extra time is needed during an examination. However, the employer cannot probe and ask: How long have you had epilepsy? How many medications do you take? or other such questions.

Medical Examinations

The ADA's rules about medical exams differ depending upon the employment status of the individual. *Before* offering a job, employers are not allowed to conduct any type of medical examination. *After* a conditional offer of employment, the ADA allows employers to require medical examinations of its employees if routine for all employees in that particular job. If a disability such as epilepsy is disclosed during the medical interviews and examination, it is confidential (except for first aid and safety personnel) and cannot be used to refuse employment if essential job functions can be performed.

Testing for Illegal Drugs

Employers can test for illegal drugs during any stage of the application process or during employment, if all employees are required to take a drug test as part of company policy. The employer cannot use the results of a drug test to discriminate against a disabled person taking prescribed medication.

Explaining Seizures to Coworkers

A person with epilepsy whose seizures are not well controlled should prepare for the possibility that a seizure may occur at work. The preparation will depend on the type and frequency of seizures. First, discuss the seizures with the supervisor and coworkers. They will be the first ones to see the seizure and to administer first aid. Depending on the work environment, the people, the relationships with coworkers, and the nature of the seizures, a person with epilepsy may choose to tell only a few people =or everyone. Never rely entirely on one coworker, however, because that person may be on vacation or out of the office when a seizure occurs.

It is often a good idea to review first aid measures in a group setting. Others in the workplace need to know what happens during a seizure and what to do. The explanation should be reassuring. First aid cards, videos (epilepsy.com), and other educational materials can help.

Vocational Rehabilitation

Vocational rehabilitation services can help those who have never held a job or who have been out of the work force to train for and get employment that meets their individual needs. It provides specialized training to help them develop skills, confidence, and strategies to help make up for problems and enhance their chances for employment.

The Rehabilitation Act of 1973 provides employment rights for people with disabilities. Many vocational rehabilitation services are available that address a range of needs. These services *may* include, but are not limited to:

- *Diagnostic evaluation* to assess any disability and determine eligibility and to help establish a career development plan

- *Counseling* to set goals, make choices, determine job-skill training needed, and provide support

>⊛ *Psychological, physical,* or *occupational therapies*

>⊛ *Training* to teach job skills, compensatory, job search strategies, interviewing skills and job coaching, resume writing, and legal rights

>⊛ Referral to training programs

>⊛ *Transportation*

>⊛ *Job placement* in the competitive work force, in supported community employment or in sheltered workshops, or in the home

>⊛ *Postemployment* services to help employees keep their jobs, and job accommodation assistance

Individualized Written Rehabilitation Plan

The vocational rehabilitation counselor helps to develop an individualized written rehabilitation plan that identifies the goals, services, and goods needed for employment. The disabled person may be joined by a parent, guardian, or someone else.

Workers' Compensation

Every state has laws that guarantee compensation for job-related injuries. Employers must either be self-insured or insured through the state workers' compensation program. Work-related injuries are only covered if the injury occurred during work (not while going to or from work) and was clearly a result of the employment. Therefore, if someone with epilepsy falls at work and is injured the accident is usually not covered. However, work-related factors could cause or contribute to seizure-related injuries. For example, excessive overtime and stress can lead to sleep deprivation or exhaustion.

Military Service

The United States armed services (Army, Navy, Air Force, Coast Guard, and state National Guard) require that members be available for duty 24 hours a day and have no condition that could impair their performance under adverse conditions. Because sleep deprivation and lack of medication can cause seizures in people with epilepsy, there are strict regulations regarding the enlistment of people with epilepsy.

Currently, the armed services require those enlisting to be seizure-free without medications for at least 5 years. Cases are reviewed on an individual basis, and an appeal can be made for those who have been seizure-free for a shorter period, depending on their medical history, prognosis, and the specific position they seek.

Persons with any disorder that can cause a sudden loss of consciousness or motor control are excluded from flight training. The only exception is for individuals who had febrile seizures before age 5 and now have a normal EEG.

When a member of the armed services develops seizures or epilepsy, he or she may be discharged because of the disorder, but the regulations do not require automatic dismissal unless the person's seizures are not fully controlled by AEDs.

29 | Epilepsy in the Elderly

Epilepsy can begin at any age, and the rate of newly diagnosed epilepsy is higher in elderly people than in middle-aged adults. As in younger people, the cause of epilepsy often cannot be determined when it begins in the elderly. Approximately half of the cases are caused by stroke (often a small one that did not cause other symptoms), head injury, or tumor (either benign or malignant). Recurrent seizures may also be caused by metabolic disorders or drugs (prescribed, over-the-counter, alcohol). Degenerative disorders such as Alzheimer's disease are a rare cause of seizures in the elderly.

Effects of Seizures on Older People

There are special concerns about the effects of seizures on older people. The body becomes less resilient with age, so the effects of tonic-clonic seizures can cause more serious damage. They can stress the heart and lungs and cause potential problems for people with cardiac or pulmonary disorders. Similarly, breathing is affected during a tonic-clonic seizure, which can aggravate lung disorders. Bones also are more fragile, increasing the risk of fracture during a tonic-clonic seizure or seizure-related fall. Despite these and other potential problems, most older people who suffer tonic-clonic seizures have no serious aftereffects. Postictal states of tiredness, weakness, cognitive impairment, or behavioral change can be more severe and prolonged in older individuals. When the weakness is on one side, a stroke may be misdiagnosed.

Effects of AEDs and Other Medications on the Elderly

A 74-year-old woman began to experience twitching movements on the right side of her face. A CT scan showed a benign tumor—a meningioma—on the surface of the left frontal lobe. She was treated with phenytoin, and the seizures stopped. The tumor was surgically removed. She had no seizures for 6 months after the operation while taking phenytoin (400 mg) in the morning, but then the twitching movements returned. Most of the twitching movements occurred in the late evening or would awaken her from sleep. Around lunch, she was tired and unsteady, which she attributed to the drug.

Her doctor increased the dose to 500 mg a day, but side effects increased. Two months later, her internist prescribed sucralfate (Carafate) for a stomach problem, and she had a brief tonic-clonic seizure during sleep several weeks later. The blood phenytoin level early in the morning, before she took her pills, was low; around lunch the level was high. The phenytoin was divided into two doses and eventually adjusted to 200 mg in the morning and 230 mg at night. Sucralfate, which can lower phenytoin levels, was discontinued, and another medication that did not interact was prescribed. The phenytoin level became much steadier, the side effects almost completely disappeared, and the seizures were fully controlled.

This case report illustrates several important aspects of therapy for epilepsy in older patients. People become more sensitive to the effects of medications as they grow older. This woman experienced side effects when the blood phenytoin level was in the therapeutic range, common for many older people on many AEDs and other medications. Older people (and sometimes younger ones) may need to go on a twice-a-day (or more frequent) regimen of phenytoin or other AEDs to "smooth out" their blood levels, thereby reducing the chances of both seizures and side effects. Drug interactions also can be a problem, especially in the elderly who, on average, are taking more than three drugs. The doctor should be informed of all prescription and over-the-counter medications the patient is taking.

Some medications often used to treat the elderly may provoke seizures. These medications include drugs used to treat behavioral and psychiatric problems, asthma, heart disorders, and infections. Therefore, all persons with epilepsy or with a history of epilepsy should inform their doctors, because a medication prescribed for an unrelated problem could make seizures more likely.

Which antiepileptic drugs is the best one for the elderly to take?

There is no "best" drug. A large controlled study compared carbamazepine, gabapentin, and lamotrigine in the elderly. All three drugs were equally effective, but the lamotrigine caused the fewest side effects; gabapentin was intermediate, and carbamazepine caused the most side effects. Levetiracetam, which has no drug interactions and does not induce liver enzymes or cause bone loss, is also effective and well tolerated in low doses by elderly people.

V

Legal and Financial Issues in Epilepsy

30 | Legal Rights of People with Epilepsy

U nfortunately, discrimination against people with disabilities, especially epilepsy, continues in employment, public accommodations, and housing. State and federal government protects people with disabilities against discrimination. However, people with epilepsy may face unjust accusation of antisocial or criminal behavior after a seizure in public, illegal denial of adequate medical care in correctional facilities, and problems in child adoption or child custody cases.

Medical Care

In the United States, no one has a legal right to medical care. However, most hospital emergency departments do not refuse medical care to someone who has a serious medical problem. The greatest problem for many people is availability of medical insurance. Individuals and families whose income is low but exceeds a certain amount may apply for Medicaid benefits (see Chapter 31). Some states also provide health care to all children.

Public Services

Some state laws protecting the rights of people with disabilities are extensions to their civil rights laws, and others are part of a comprehensive handicap discrimination law. In some states, protection against discrimination for people with disabilities extends to services rendered by, regulated by, or funded by the state. Thus, state laws may also provide protection in areas such as education, insurance, licensing, and access to transportation.

Public Accommodations

Rarely, someone with epilepsy is unfairly prohibited from entering public places such as a hotel or restaurant. The ADA prohibits places of public accommodation (excluding religious organizations and private clubs) from discriminating against individuals with disabilities.

Housing

The Fair Housing Amendments Act (FHAA) of 1988 prohibits discrimination in the sale, rental, or financing of housing because of a disability. The FHAA mandates that housing providers make "reasonable accommodations" in rules, policies, and services to allow people with disabilities equal opportunities.

Airline Travel

People with epilepsy can be passengers on airplanes, because there is no evidence that seizures are more likely to occur during or shortly after airplane flights than at other times. For those who have uncontrolled seizures, it may be worthwhile considering special precautions. If the person is traveling alone, inform flight attendants about the disorder so they respond appropriately. If a tonic-clonic seizure occurs in someone without a known history of epilepsy, the airline may divert a coast-to-coast flight to have the person treated in a city en route.

False Arrest

After complex partial or tonic-clonic seizures, people are often confused and may appear to be under the influence of alcohol or illegal drugs.

In this setting, persons with epilepsy may be unfairly arrested and charged. During complex partial seizures, some persons may perform automatic acts that are misinterpreted as willful and criminal. For example, they may undress in public, grab someone's arm, or pick up something in a store and break it or place it in a pocket. In these cases, a careful description of the act; the person's behavior before, during, and after the behavior; and a statement from family members or friends of the person's behavior during previous seizures can be extremely helpful. Unfortunately, a person's first seizure may be the one for which he or she is unjustly accused of criminal behavior. A doctor can usually determine if the behavior occurred during or after a seizure, and a doctor's report can lead to dismissal of the charges.

Restraint after seizures should be avoided, as even relatively mild restraint can lead to violent reactions. During and after a seizure that impairs consciousness, the confused person may misinterpret physical contact and may respond in an aggressive manner. The person with epilepsy can then be charged with assault or resisting arrest or be injured by law enforcement officers or others. In the worst case, seizures and their aftereffects are mistaken for criminal behavior, and the person with epilepsy is jailed, denied medication, and suffers additional seizures.

Wearing a bracelet or necklace (or, less so, carrying a card in a wallet) that identifies someone as having epilepsy can avoid mistreatment and possible unjust arrest. The bracelet or necklace should have the diagnosis, medications, and telephone numbers of their doctor and the person to call in case of an emergency. In addition, when traveling, people with epilepsy should carry their medications in the bottle from the pharmacy or carry a copy of the prescription or a doctor's note.

Child Adoption

Persons with epilepsy can adopt children. Laws concerning adoption are generally written with safeguards to ensure the child's best interests. The fitness of a potential adoptive parent may be questioned because he or she has seizures. Many states require consideration of the mental and physical health of prospective parents. If the seizures are fully or partially controlled, there should be no restrictions.

Child Custody

Persons with epilepsy can obtain custody of their children. Courts deciding custody matters should primarily consider the best interests of the child. A parent's epilepsy should not affect most custody decisions. Case law states that epilepsy should not be the sole basis for denying custody to a parent, but can be considered in determining the child's best interests.

For a parent whose seizures are completely or partially controlled, the custody decision should not be influenced by epilepsy. Unfortunately, negative attitudes toward epilepsy still persist, and some courts may unfairly deny custody on the basis of perceptions, not facts.

The parent with epilepsy should be ready to provide detailed information about the type, duration, and frequency of seizures and about medications taken. If the seizures impair consciousness or control of movement, it may help to discuss specific safeguards to protect the child. If the other spouse claims that the child was injured during a seizure in the parent with epilepsy, the event should be carefully investigated and the direct relevance of the seizure examined. The claim may be made that seizures will psychologically harm the child; there is no evidence to support this claim!

If epilepsy was a factor in making a custody decision, and the disorder later comes under better control, the parent should present a doctor's statement of the improvement and request a change in the custody decision.

31 | Insurance and Government Assistance for People with Epilepsy

People with epilepsy need to be concerned about health insurance as well as life insurance, mortgage insurance, and disability insurance to provide security for themselves and their families. In addition to the financial protection afforded by private insurance, the federal government offers health insurance to people who meet certain eligibility requirements—the Medicare and Medicaid programs. These types of federal insurance and income maintenance programs are also available to those who qualify.

Health Insurance

Lack of affordable health care remains a serious problem. Health care costs are increasing and private health insurance moves further from the reach of many. Health insurance policies are expensive, especially for people with preexisting conditions such as epilepsy. People with epilepsy who have health insurance may find that certain diagnostic procedures and treatments are not covered or difficult to get approved. For example, some plans make the patient and referring doctor "jump through hoops" to authorize specialized services (such as video-EEG monitoring). The insurer's approval can often be obtained if both the patient and the doctor persist in documenting the need for specialized services.

There are different categories of health insurance. Commercial or private indemnity insurance policies are the most expensive, but provide the most comprehensive coverage. They allow the patient to choose the doctor and hospital. These plans typically pay all or a large portion of hospital, outpatient test, and doctor bills.

Health maintenance organizations (HMOs) and preferred provider organizations (PPOs) are health care systems formed by groups of doctors and hospitals. Medical care is usually rendered only by the individuals and institutions within the system. In these organizations, as well as managed health care plans (see below), a single doctor may act as a "gatekeeper." He or she must approve all tests and referrals to other doctors within or outside the group. Usually no fee or only a small fee is charged for medical services. These organizations can limit the number of diagnostic procedures.

Managed group health care plans are also becoming more common. These plans often use a large network of doctors, laboratories, community hospitals, and university-related medical centers. The picture is becoming even more complex, as many managed health care companies include their traditional plans, point-of-service plans, HMOs, PPOs, Medicare+Choice plans, and third-party administration of employer-funded benefit plans.

Group health plans may offer greater protection for people with epilepsy because of the Health Insurance Portability and Accountability Act (HIPAA) of 1996. This act requires that group health plans cannot exclude a preexisting condition from coverage for more than 12 months, provided the condition is one that is generally covered in the policy.

The Comprehensive Omnibus Benefits Reform Act (COBRA) of 1984, a federal law, helps people maintain insurance coverage when they leave group health plans. Persons who are no longer eligible for group health coverage can purchase COBRA coverage for up to 18 months. COBRA and HIPAA can work together to (1) maintain coverage while a person finds or starts a new job and (2) limit the exclusion period for a preexisting condition that may apply to a new insurance plan.

Medicare

Medicare, administered by the federal Health Care Financing Administration, is health insurance for all members of our society aged

65 or over and for people who receive Social Security Disability Insurance (SSDI) benefits for at least 2 years. Medicare benefits are divided into two parts: Part A and Part B. Part A covers hospital services and skilled nursing services, except for a modest deductible paid by the patient. Part B covers doctor services, some home health services, outpatient hospital services such as physical and occupational therapies, and nondisposable equipment. Most people with Medicare can pay a monthly premium to help lower prescription drug costs.

Medicaid

Medicaid, a federal-state program administered by the states, provides health insurance to individuals over 65 years of age and people with disabilities who meet specific income and medical criteria. Eligibility and benefits vary from state to state. Most states provide coverage for hospital and doctor services; inpatient and outpatient services and prescription drugs are usually included. In many states, a person who is eligible for Supplemental Security Income (SSI) is automatically eligible for Medicaid.

The majority of private practice ("fee-for-service") doctors do not accept Medicaid, whose reimbursement often does not cover the expenses for maintaining the office (rent, utilities, staff, malpractice insurance). However, many teaching hospitals and epilepsy centers have clinics that accept Medicaid.

Life Insurance

Epilepsy can influence a person's eligibility for life insurance, as well as the cost of insurance. Insurance companies rely on statistics regarding lifestyle, habits, and life span in different diseases and disorders when deciding on whether to offer life insurance and how much to charge for it. Because epilepsy does not follow the same course for everyone, it is unfair for insurance companies to lump together everyone with a history of epilepsy. Most insurance companies are aware of this and usually ask for a medical history from the doctor.

One should be honest about a history of epilepsy on a life insurance application. If the insurance company investigates after the insured person's death and finds that a disorder was concealed, the company may deny benefits, even if death was not relatedto epilepsy.

Mortgage Insurance

Mortgage insurance is a kind of life insurance. In case of the insured person's death, it will pay off the remainder of the mortgage. It provides another form of security for the family. As with life insurance, mortgage insurance can be more difficult to obtain and more expensive for people with epilepsy.

Disability Insurance

For people younger than 45 years old, chances are greater that they will be disabled than that they will die. People whose income is critical for their own support or their family's support should consider disability insurance. Unfortunately, it is expensive and gets more expensive as a person gets older. People with epilepsy may find disability insurance difficult to obtain and expensive because some of them have a greater chance of becoming disabled.

Government Financial Assistance

Social Security Disability Benefits

The federal government's Social Security Administration (SSA) sponsors two programs that provide monthly income payments to individuals whose disabilities are expected to prevent them from working for at least 12 months. Disability is defined by the inability of the person "to engage in any substantial gainful activity by reason of any medically determinable physical or mental impairment which can be expected to result in death or which has lasted or can be expected to last for a continuous period of not less than 12 months."

Establishing eligibility for Social Security disability benefits can be a difficult process. Criteria are strictly enforced, and many deserving applicants are initially denied benefits but later approved on appeal. Persons can file an appeal with an attorney. If the appeal is successful, payments are retroactive to the date of the initial application.

The first program, Social Security Disability Insurance (SSDI), pays benefits to eligible workers under age 65 (and their dependents or survivors) who have worked for a minimum period and have paid Social Security taxes.

The second program, Supplemental Security Income (SSI), is based on need and does not require prior payment of Social Security taxes. To qualify, the applicant must have limited assets (cash or other property), and the monthly income cannot exceed a certain amount per month. (See www.ssa.gov or call 1-800-772-1213.) Disabled children under age 18 years who live at home are considered to have their parents' income and assets and are therefore usually not eligible for SSI, but special rules apply to some children.

Social Security Administration Criteria for Eligibility

The SSA considers epileptic seizures in two broad groups:

- *Major motor:* tonic-clonic (grand mal)

- *Minor motor:* absence (petit mal), complex partial (psychomotor), and focal motor

Major motor seizures must occur at least once a month despite at least 3 months of treatment. There must be either daytime seizures with loss of consciousness or convulsive seizures, or seizures during sleep with residual effects that interfere significantly with daytime function. Minor motor seizures must occur more often than once a week despite at least 3 months of treatment. There must be "alteration of awareness or loss of consciousness and transient postictal manifestations of unconventional behavior or significant interference with activity during the day."

If epilepsy causes the disability, the SSA requires documentation of the disorder with an EEG and a detailed description of a typical seizure. A written diary recording the date and time of seizures, medication changes, and side effects can help document the seizure history. SSA recognizes that a normal EEG does not rule out the diagnosis of epilepsy. Detailed documentation of a typical seizure is essential.

The description should include whether or not there is a warning or an aura (and its features), tongue biting, loss of bladder or bowel control, injuries caused by the seizure, and postseizure symptoms such as confusion or sleepiness. The doctor's description of the seizure should state the source of the information and whether corroboration was obtained. If a health professional witnessed a seizure, those observations should be included. The SSA may to request that the applicant see an agency-paid doctor.

Several other issues may be relevant to the determination of disability benefits on the basis of epilepsy:

- Although the actual seizure count for the last 2 months may not fulfill the SSA criteria, the average seizure frequency over the past 6–12 months can be used, because seizures often occur in clusters. This point must be emphasized, as a cluster of three seizures in 2 days can be extremely disabling. Although this criterion is not yet recognized, it could be argued that this seizure frequency is equivalent to the one currently used and has a similar meaning for determining the presence of a disability.

- If seizures can only be controlled with very high dosages of medications, then the disabling effects of these drugs must also be considered.

- Documentation of AED blood levels can confirm that he or she takes the prescribed medications. If the levels are below the therapeutic range even though the medication is being taken as prescribed, then the person's doctor should note that the low levels may be due to problems with absorption or rapid metabolism or to the person's inability to tolerate higher levels because of side effects.

Returning to Work

Under the Ticket to Work and Work Incentives Improvement Act, government financial assistance and health benefits (such as Medicare or Medicaid) can continue for a limited time even after a disabled person returns to work. Many people receiving SSDI can keep full benefits for as long as 1 year after they return to work.

VI

Resources for People with Epilepsy

32 | Mental Health of Adults with Epilepsy

P eople with epilepsy are often subject to depression, anxiety, irritability, and more serious mental disorders. The psychiatric problems may be unrelated to epilepsy or may be related to the person's emotional reactions to having epilepsy, the effect of medications, the underlying cause of epilepsy (such as scar tissue from head trauma), or the epilepsy itself.

Behavioral changes can occur around the time of a seizure (peri-ictal) or during the idnterval between seizures (interictal). Peri-ictal changes can occur before (preictal), during (ictal), or after (postictal) a seizure. Some individuals and family members report premonitory symptoms such as irritability or sadness occurring hours or even days before a seizure. Emotions are common during partial seizures, with negative feelings such as fear and anxiety most common (see Chapter 2). After a complex partial or tonic-clonic seizure, people may experience depression, irritability, anxiety, or mania. After a prolonged or cluster of complex partial or tonic-clonic seizures, behavioral changes can be more pronounced and occasionally include psychosis. Most of the behavioral changes discussed below occur interictally—between seizures. These are sustained and relatively stable patterns of behavior.

Personality Changes

Throughout history, a variety of derogatory labels have been applied to the personalities of people with epilepsy. Many neurologists once believed that there was an "epileptic personality." Although studies show that some people with epilepsy may undergo personality changes, the frequency, severity, and negativity of these changes has often been exaggerated.

Certain behavioral traits may be more common in people with epilepsy than in the general population. These include increased emotionality, irritability, "social clinginess" (a tendency towards prolonged interpersonal contact), circumlocution (talking around a point), excessive writing (hypergraphia), greater than usualreligiousness or moral or philosophical interests, a sense of personal destiny, altered sexual interest (usually decreased libido), irritability, and anger. They are not specific for people with epilepsy and are also more frequent among people with some psychiatric and other disorders than among the general public.

Controversy continues as to whether certain traits are more frequent in people with temporal lobe epilepsy than in those with other forms of partial epilepsy or generalized epilepsy. Since the temporal and frontal lobes both contain limbic areas that control emotional and social functions, as well as other areas that determine executive (judgment, reasoning) and personality (especially frontal lobe) functions, any disorder (head trauma, epilepsy, stroke, etc) affecting these areas could potentially alter behavior.

Generalized epilepsies, such as absence and juvenile myoclonic epilepsy, are also associated with an increased frequency of psychiatric disorders such as depression and anxiety. The generalized epilepsies, although they are fundamentally different from partial epilepsies, also affect frontal (mainly) and temporal regions, as well as other cortical and subcortical regions. A well-designed study compared children with absence epilepsy to those with juvenile rheumatoid arthritis (which controls for the effects of chronic illness) at a follow-up after age 18. Those with absence epilepsy had greater difficulties with academic, personal, and behavioral functioning.

The study of personality and epilepsy has raised more questions than it has answered. Although personality changes and disorders are more frequent among people with epilepsy than in the general population, the causes remain uncertain. The relative roles of epilepsy, psychological response to epilepsy, genetics, family and socioeconomic background, medications, brain abnormalities that cause epilepsy, and other factors remain uncertain. When personality or behavioral changes interfere with personal, family, or professional life, help should be sought.

Depression

Depression causes feelings of sadness, helplessness, hopelessness, and guilt and impairs a person's ability to experience happiness. Other problems include difficulty with sleeping (insomnia or sleeping excessively), decreased sexual desire, and appetite disturbances (loss of appetite or overeating).

Depression is common in the general population, but it occurs more often in those who have epilepsy. The depth and duration of sadness that affects most people varies considerably. The borderline between sadness and depression is not precise, but when sadness is prolonged and impairs a person's ability to enjoy life and to work, there is a problem.

The most serious complication of depression is suicide. The rate of suicide is increased in people with epilepsy. Patients, family members, and doctors often fail to recognize the presence or severity of depression. If there is any question, seek help. Anyone who expresses thoughts about hurting himself or herself should be taken extremely seriously. If someone who is depressed discusses a specific plan to hurt him- or herself or gives away treasured items, a psychiatrist should be consulted *immediately*.

Causes of Depression

Depression can result from a psychological reaction to having epilepsy; from medication effects; from the cause of the epilepsy, such as head injury or stroke; or from the epilepsy itself. The relative importance of each of these factors varies in each case, and often several factors contribute. In some cases the depression is related to loss of a job or a loved one or to a flurry of seizures. Depression related to the psychological effects of living with epilepsy often improves by discussing troublesome feelings with a therapist.

AEDs, especially barbiturates (phenobarbital and primidone), can cause depression. This kind of depression is often dose-related; that is, the higher the dose, the greater the risk and severity of depression. Taking one or more other AEDs in combination with a barbiturate can also increase the risk. If a depressed person takes a barbiturate, he or she should ask the doctor about a medication change. Other AEDs, especially benzodiazepines, levetiracetam, topiramate, and vigabatrin, also can also contribute to or cause depression in some people. Other medications such as beta-blockers and steroids can also cause depression.

Treatment of Depression

When possible, the cause or causes of the depression should be treated. Serious depression requires antidepressant medication. Some doctors fear that antidepressants can aggravate the seizure disorder, but several studies suggest that patients are more likely to have improved seizure control, possibly by improving mood and restorative sleep and reducing stress. Newer antidepressants such as the selective serotonin reuptake inhibitors (SSRIs) appear safe for almost all epilepsy patients. These drugs include fluoxetine (Prozac), paroxetine (Paxil), sertraline (Zoloft), citalopram (Celexa), and escitalopram (Lexapro). Other antidepressant drugs that are safe for most patients with epilepsy include venlafaxine (Effexor) and duloxetine (Cymbalta), which inhibit reuptake of serotonin and norepinephrines. These "serotonin" drugs also can help treat obsessive-compulsive disorder and anxiety disorder. Bupropion is used to treat depression (Wellbutrin) and help people to stop smoking (Zyban). Initial experience with high doses of buproprion (450 mg/day) suggested that seizures were a common side effect. However, greater experience with other populations and doses of up to 300 mg/day suggests the risk of provoking a seizure or exacerbating epilepsy is low. Very severe depression in epilepsy patients may be treated with electroconvulsive shock therapy.

Anxiety

Anxiety disorders are more common among people with epilepsy. Anxiety and nervousness become a disorder when the feelings are frequent or intense, are produced by trivial things or nothing at all, and interfere with functioning. Several factors can cause anxiety disorders, including psychological stress related to the epilepsy or other issues, medication effects, associated neurologic or psychiatric disorders, and the epilepsy itself.

Anxiety disorders can be effectively treated with counseling, therapy, and medications. Buspirone (Buspar) is safe for almost all patients with epilepsy and anxiety. The SSRIs, listed in the section on depression, also can help treat anxiety.

Benzodiazepines are very effective in the short-term treatment of anxiety and insomnia, but they should be avoided if possible because they are among the most habit-forming (addictive) drugs legally available. Benzodiazepines commonly used to treat anxiety include clonazepam (Klonopin), diazepam (Valium), alprazolam (Xanax), clorazepate (Tranxene), and lorazepam (Ativan). These drugs also may temporarily reduce seizure frequency and intensity, but after a period of weeks, the effect on anxiety, insomnia, and seizure control diminishes. As the original anxiety or seizures return, there is a strong tendency for the patient and doctor to increase the dose, which again briefly reduces troublesome symptoms. This cycle leads to a build-up of the dose to levels that can cause memory impairment, depression, tiredness, and other problems. If the dose is then reduced, the real trouble begins: anxiety, insomnia, and seizures become more severe.

Irritability

People with epilepsy may be more prone toward irritability. In addition to stress and tiredness, irritability may also be related to medications, especially the barbiturates (but also levetiracetam, zonisamide, and others), to brain abnormalities in areas that regulate emotions, and the epilepsy itself. Irritability may precede or follow seizures.

A change in medications or improved seizure control may reduce anxiety and irritability. For the few people with epilepsy in whom irritability is a serious problem, discuss it with the doctor. A change in AED or dosage, treatment of an underlying depression or sleep disorder, or psychotherapy may be beneficial. Buspirone (Buspar) and SSRIs (see above) can also help. In more serious cases, low doses of antipsychotic medications may be used.

Psychosis

Psychosis is a serious mental disorder with impaired content and coherence of thoughts, reduced connection to reality, and paranoia. The person may experience delusions or disturbances of perception (hallucinations and distortions of sensation) or extremes of emotions. The person may display decreased drive and motivation, social withdrawal and detachment, or either hyperactivity or immobility. In some cases, the person may harm themself or others.

Psychosis can be a purely psychiatric disorder without any associated neurologic disorder (as in schizophrenia). Psychosis can also result from brain injuries, or it can be caused by certain medications such as amphetamines (stimulants). Persons with epilepsy have an increased rate of interictal psychosis (psychosis "in between" seizures, not only around the time of seizures). Patients with temporal lobe epilepsy appear to be at the greatest risk.

Psychosis can develop after seizures, usually after a cluster of complex partial or tonic-clonic seizures. These individuals often appear well for a few hours or days and then express disordered thoughts, delusional ideas (for example, paranoid thoughts that someone is going to hurt him or her), and aggressive behavior. Such psychoses are usually relatively brief and can be effectively treated with medications (antipsychotic drugs and benzodiazepines). Prompt recognition and treatment of this disorder are most important.

Newer antipsychotic drugs are safe for people with epilepsy. These drugs include quetiapine (Seroquel), rispiridone (Risperidal), olanzapine (Zyprexa), aripiprazole (Abilify), and ziprasidone (Geodon).

Aggression

The stigmatizing relation of epilepsy and aggressive behavior was exaggerated in the past. Some children and adults with epilepsy show aggressive behavior that may be related to antiepileptic drugs, underlying brain abnormalities, epilepsy, or the confused (postictal) state after seizures. The vast majority of people with epilepsy are no more likely to be aggressive or commit a violent crime than anyone else in the general population.

Children have less impulse control than adults. They translate thoughts into actions more readily. Control over social behavior and aggressive impulses is acquired relatively late in childhood as the brain develops and matures. Some children with epilepsy, and those with other neurologic disorders such as mental retardation, have higher rates of aggressive behaviors than other children. In part, this results from dysfunction in brain areas that control social behavior and impulses. Similar aggressive behaviors may develop in adults after brain such as head trauma, even if they have never had a seizure.

Certain medications can make aggressive behavior more likely to occur, especially in predisposed individuals. The barbiturates (phenobarbital and primidone) are most likely to cause aggressive behaviors. Although barbiturates usually havetranquilizing effects, they can cause agitation. Other AEDs and some stimulants, such as dextroamphetamine, also can trigger aggressive behaviors.

During a complex partial seizure, directed aggressive behavior is exceedingly rare. Aggressive behavior can occur during the period of confusion after a tonic-clonic seizure, usually because someone tries to restrain the person. The best response to such a reaction is to remove the restraint.

Unusual Seizures

Some persons with epilepsy, especially those with partial seizures, may experience unusual and bizarre phenomena during seizures. The experiences can be fascinating, frightening, or both. Very often, people are reluctant to discuss strange symptoms or experiences for fear of being considered odd or crazy. However, symptoms that begin suddenly and last for a brief time can be a seizure, no matter how strange they seem.

The following are descriptions of unusual seizures, often provided only after specific questions were asked:

> I had a feeling of extreme embarrassment, as though I had made a very foolish remark.

I feel that someone else is in the room behind me.

Looking into the mirror, I noticed that the right side of my face was missing.

On the left half of space there were colored balls of light. As I looked at them, they changed to multiple figures of small men. On later occasions, I recognized these as myself—tiny replicas that would approach and then recede.

I have a flood of thoughts; I don't know where they come from; I can't shut them off.

Scenes appear in my mind's eye. I have never lived them, they must be imaginary, but they appear real. I sort of know what is going on around me, but I am also a bit tuned out.

My seizures start with a warning of fear, and then I feel as if I am a character in the PacMan video game and the monster is going to eat me. I am actually in the machine.

It is the most frightening feeling, as if I know the worst thing in the world is about to happen, I just don't know what.

> The next thing I knew I was floating just below the ceiling. I could see myself lying there. I wasn't scared; it was too interesting. Next I was in space and could see the Earth.

These experiences are not typical seizure symptoms. The range of seizure symptoms is extremely broad; almost any emotion or experience is possible. Although most seizure symptoms are brief, lasting less than 3 minutes—on rare occasions they can last more than 10 or 15 minutes. The important feature is the sudden onset, although symptoms and experiences unrelated to epilepsy can also begin suddenly.

Patients who experience phenomena such as the ones described should mention them to their doctor. If the symptoms precede definite complex partial or tonic-clonic seizures, they very likely are part of the seizure (a simple partial seizure).

33 | Resources for People with Epilepsy

The Internet

The Internet is the most powerful source for information and communication. For people with epilepsy and their families, it is *the* place to learn and share experiences. Yet it is a two-sided coin—much information is reliable and accurate, and much is inaccurate and misleading. Be wary of sites that promote products or services. Start with an established, noncommercial website: epilepsy.com is my recommendation for an overall outstanding place to begin. Other excellent sites include epilepsyfoundation.org (see below), aesnet.org (American Epilepsy Society site; their information on antiepileptic drugs and the journal *Epilepsy Currents* is very informative), epilepsy.org (International League Against Epilepsy and International Bureau for Epilepsy), comprehensive epilepsy center sites, and PubMed (cbi.nlm.nih.gov/entrez/; an excellent place to search for abstracts on scientific articles).

Epilepsy.com

Epilepsy.com provides in-depth information and a community to educate and empower patients, families, and caregivers living with epilepsy. The site is supported by the nonprofit Epilepsy Therapy Project (see Chapter 34) and addresses a wide spectrum of needs, from those newly diagnosed with epilepsy to those living with epilepsy that has resisted treatment. Epilepsy.com provides accessible written and multimedia content including Epilepsy 101, an overview of epilepsy and seizures and available therapies, and offers the most in-depth information available on the web on epilepsy therapies.

The epilepsy.com community includes a broad range of discussion threads, blogs, and chat including People Stories and commentary on living with epilepsy. The clinical trial listings offer a comprehensive source for locating all clinical trials ongoing in epilepsy. News and articles reporting on emerging therapies and standards of care are provided by the editorial board, consisting of leading epileptologists and experts.

Seizure preparedness and first aid and the needs of specialized populations including women, children, teens, and men are each addressed in individual sections. An online seizure diary and medical management tool helps individuals and caregivers manage their seizures and medications and communicate with their doctors and other caregivers. The Pipeline Update looks at new therapies under development.

Epilepsy.com brings together reliable insights from experts with user-generated content capturing the real world experience of the broad community of doctors and nurses who treat epilepsy and of the families who live with it. The result is relevant—lively information, discussion, and community focused on the best available therapies for living well with epilepsy.

The Epilepsy Foundation

The Epilepsy Foundation is the national voluntary health organization committed to the prevention and cure of seizure disorders, the easing of their effects, and the promotion of independence and the best possible quality of life for people with these disorders.

Programs and Activities

The Epilepsy Foundation supports programs at the national and local levels to improve the lives of people with epilepsy and their families. The foundation has affiliates in most states. The affiliates are independently organized state and local groups that are bound to the national organization by an affiliation agreement.

The national office of the Epilepsy Foundation works with its affiliates to provide local services and a variety of educational, research, legislative, and other programs. The programs offered by the affiliates varies depending on local needs and support.

Information and Referral Services

The national Epilepsy Foundation office offers a toll-free number (800-332-1000) to provide information and referrals. The foundation provides information on a wide range of epilepsy-related topics and on local resources. The Epilepsy Foundation's affiliates also distribute information about epilepsy and local services. Referrals to local medical, psychological, social, and other services can be provided.

Information and Education

The Epilepsy Foundation produces and distributes educational materials about epilepsy, including pamphlets, videotapes, posters, and books. More than 30 pamphlets cover topics such as basic information, medicines, legal rights and issues, employment, first aid for seizures, information for babysitters of children with epilepsy, parenting children with epilepsy, and epilepsy and learning disabilities.

The Internet

The Epilepsy Foundation's website (www.epilepsyfoundation.org) offers information for individuals, families, and the general public to learn more about seizure disorders.

Advocacy Programs

The foundation's advocacy program helps fight discrimination; promotes access to health care, education, and employment; and supports independent living. Representatives testify in support of essential government programs related to the needs of people with epilepsy. These include medical research, improved quality of medical care, better access to insurance, financial assistance for the disabled and ill, and employment and rehabilitation programs. Legal advocacy is another important program.

Employment Programs

Local affiliates may provide job counseling, job clubs, employer outreach services to improve opportunities, and other services.

National Conference

The foundation's annual conference brings together volunteers and staff of its local affiliates, national staff, health care professionals, people with epilepsy, and their families. Each conference has a theme and includes lectures and workshops.

Counseling Programs and Support Groups

Professionally staffed counseling programs or peer group support programs involving people with epilepsy or their parents are offered by many of the affiliates. Counseling sessions may cover such issues as adjusting to and living with epilepsy and parenting a child with epilepsy. Support groups allow people to gain strength from shared experiences.

School Alert

The School Alert programs are local programs to improve the school environment for children with epilepsy. Information about epilepsy is made available to teachers, school nurses, other school personnel, and students through videotapes, manuals, pamphlets, and in-person presentations of the Epilepsy Foundation's curriculum on seizure recognition and first aid. For young children, the "Kids on the Block" puppet show is offered by many affiliates to present the information in a child-friendly way.

Camping Programs

Many affiliates offer camping experiences, often combined with epilepsy education, for children with epilepsy. Parents whose children go to these camps frequently find they are more independent and self-confident afterward.

Respite Care

When a child has severe seizures or associated disabilities, parents need an occasional time out. Some affiliates offer respite care in the form of trained people to relieve parents and other family members for predetermined periods of time.

Community Resources

People, organizations, agencies, and other resources available at state or local levels can provide information, advocacy, and services to people with epilepsy and their family members. In many cases, the greatest challenge is identifying these resources. The resources range from financial assistance for food, shelter, and medical care to respite care programs for parents with severely disabled children. Some important local resources are listed below.

State Department of Education

The state department of education oversees education for all children in the state and can provide information about special education programs and services. This office can also determine help if a child is receiving the needed services to which he or she is entitled.

Board of Education

Each school district has a board of education that sets local policies and coordinates special education and other programs.

Office of Vocational Education for Handicapped Students

Information about programs for children with disabilities can be obtained from the office of vocational education.

Protection and Advocacy Offices for Individuals with Disabilities

The protection and advocacy office (the title varies between states) can provide information on the state's services for people with disabilities, which may include education, recreational activities, respite programs, residential housing, and legal representation.

Developmental Disabilities Agency

The state developmental disabilities agency allocates federal funds to nonprofit private and public organizations to assist people with developmental disabilities. Some of the services include medical care (evaluation, diagnosis, and treatment), information, social services, protection, social activities, group homes, and advocacy.

State Vocational Rehabilitation Agency

The state vocational rehabilitation agency has numerous local offices that coordinate medical, physical, and occupational therapy, and provide planning, education, and vocational programs to assist people in obtaining employment.

Comprehensive Epilepsy Centers

For many people, the care of epilepsy involves the coordination of several disciplines and may require expertise beyond the capacity of general medical or neurologic care. Comprehensive epilepsy centers can provide expert and coordinated care.

The principal doctors at comprehensive epilepsy centers are epileptologists. They are neurologists who, after training in general neurology, complete additional training in caring for people with epilepsy. This training incorporates input from various health care workers to epilepsy-related problems. Most programs include extensive training in the interpretation of EEG and video-EEG recordings, the use of investigational drugs, and epilepsy surgery.

Who needs care at an epilepsy center?

Patients whose epilepsy is well controlled without medication side effects usually do not need care at an epilepsy center. Unfortunately, in some cases, a patient may be maintained on an older regimen of medications for decades (such as phenobarbital and phenytoin) but not recognize that there are problems due to his or her medications (bone loss, tiredness, and impaired memory).

A patient may be referred to an epilepsy center because the nature of the attack is uncertain (Is it epilepsy, or something else?), the type of epilepsy is difficult to classify (Are the seizures partial or primary generalized?), or the seizures or medication side effects persist. Referral can also be made because employment problems or social disabilities resulting from the epilepsy need expert attention or an investigational drug, epilepsy surgery, or vagus nerve stimulation is recommended. Patients may be referred by their neurologist, another doctor, or by themselves.

For some persons, a single consultation at an epilepsy center may be worthwhile. For example, a woman with epilepsy who is thinking about starting a family may benefit from speaking with an expert in epilepsy and pregnancy. Although the information provided by the woman's neurologist and the epileptologist may be quite similar, it can be comforting to hear confirmation. In other cases, new information and helpful suggestions may be provided by the epileptologist.

The most common referral to a comprehensive epilepsy center is for people with poorly controlled seizures or troublesome side effects of medications. Epilepsy centers can help optimize AED regimens and recommend changes in lifestyle to control seizures or avoid side effects. For patients with seizures that do not respond to the standard AEDs, investigational drugs (see Chapter 12) or surgery may be considered. Epilepsy centers have the greatest expertise in performing investigational drug trials, epilepsy surgery, implanting and managing vagus nerve stimulators, and studying other new therapeutic tehniques such as brain stimulation (see Chapter 13).

There are differences among epilepsy centers. Some centers care predominantly for children or adults, and others care for patients of all ages. Some centers offer only consultation with an epilepsy specialist and certain diagnostic studies such as video-EEG monitoring. Other centers conduct investigational drug trials or specialize in epilepsy surgery. The types of epilepsy surgery performed, the age of patients considered for surgery, and the costs of the surgery may vary considerably at different epilepsy centers. A list of comprehensive epilepsy centers and their services can be obtained from the Epilepsy Foundation, the National Association of Epilepsy Centers (www.naec.org), and epilepsy.com.

34 | Toward a Cure for Epilepsy

Research on epilepsy continues at academic centers and companies throughout the world. New AEDs help people with difficult-to-control seizures and provide alternatives for those suffering troublesome side effects. Diagnostic studies are more sensitive, and surgical procedures are safer and more effective than ever. We can now more precisely identify brain regions from which seizures arise and map brain areas that serve critical functions. Vagus nerve stimulation is the first new therapeutic modality for epilepsy in more than a century. New diagnostic techniques are being developed to accurately predict when seizures will occur and notify individuals that a seizure is imminent. Several new devices that directly stimulate the brain or deliver drugs to the brain are under investigation to prevent or treat seizures. Basic science studies are improving our understanding of the mechanisms leading to seizures and epilepsy. We need to translate these findings into new therapies. Cure is not around the corner, but there are promising leads to major advances.

The Promise of Neuroscience

There is an explosion of scientific information on how the individual neurons work and how they communicate in normal and diseased conditions. Research is funded through federal grants, commercial ventures, and philanthropy. Epilepsy research is active in a wide spectrum of areas, including:

- Investigating electrical and chemical changes in brain cells and chemicals associated with seizures and the tendency toward having seizures
- Mapping genes linked to epilepsy
- Exploring gene therapy for epilepsy
- Studying changes of metabolism in cells during and after seizures
- Developing electrodes and minicomputers that can predict when seizures will occur
- Developing safer and more effective antiepileptic drugs
- Advancing techniques to map areas of the brain responsible for seizures and improve epilepsy surgery
- Developing techniques to stimulate brain sites to prevent or disrupt seizures
- Transplantation of stem or fetal cells

Genetic Research

A cure for epilepsy may lie in better understanding the genetics of epilepsy. Although most forms of epilepsy are not "genetic," scores of genes directly affect brain electrical excitability, and hundreds indirectly affect these processes. Unlocking the mysteries of genes that contribute to and prevent seizures could help us develop new therapies.

Genetic research has focused on epilepsy syndromes with strong inheritance patterns. Comparing DNA samples from affected and non-affected members in a family can identify the critical gene in affected individuals. The next step is finding out what protein the gene produces for and then understanding the protein's function. About a dozen genes have been identified in specific, although relatively uncommon, epilepsy syndromes such as benign familial neonatal convulsions and generalized epilepsy febrile seizures plus (GEFS+). Most of these genes are involved in "gates" and "channels" that regulate the flow of ions (such as sodium and potassium) into and out of nerve cells, thereby affecting their electrical excitability.

There are several efforts worldwide to coordinate information from the clinical (phenomic) and genetic data from large populations with epilepsy. Many people with epilepsy may have similar abnormalities in several genes that contribute to their epilepsy and other genes that influence whether or not they respond to certain AEDs. The phenome-genome studies may identify genes that contribute to seizure susceptibility or cause epilepsy in many people. Individuals with idiopathic generalized epilepsy are especially likely to have such genes, but some probably contribute in people with partial epilepsy. These large studies will provide important repositories of information.

Another target of genetic research is to identify drugs that can counteract effects of "disease" genes. For example, if a gene produces a defective protein that is part of one of the sodium channel, it may be possible to create a drug that "fills in" for the defect or regulates the channel to compensate for the defect. Another hot area is gene therapy—actually modifying the DNA. For example, in patients with genetic forms of epilepsy, one might "splice" out bad genes and replace them with good genes. Such treatments could extend to many genetic disorders in which epilepsy commonly occurs, such as mitochondrial disorders and tuberous sclerosis. In other patients, it may be possible to insert genes that will control abnormal electrical discharges.

Finally, an unexplored area in epilepsy research is proteomics. Genes code for proteins, and once made, there are complex changes and interactions in these proteins. The way in which proteins function is fundamental in biology. A better understanding of proteomics in epilepsy patients holds promise to identify new therapeutic targets.

Seizure Detection

One of the most dangerous aspects of seizures is their unpredictability. For many patients, they can occur at any time of the day and in any setting. Although some patients have auras (simple partial seizures) or myoclonic jerks that warn them when a larger seizure is about to occur, these auras may not occur before all seizures. Unpredictability keeps many persons with epilepsy away from activities such as driving and causes injuries from falls. Changes in brain electrical activity may precede the initial symptoms of a seizure. Software programs can identify rhythmic changes on EEG recordings during the early phase of a seizure. The challenge is to identify the EEG changes that precede seizures and use them to predict when seizures are going to occur.

Several research groups are working on devices that make EEG recordings directly from the brain using electrodes implanted on top of the brain (under the skull) attached to small computers to predict when a seizure will occur. If we could reliably identify the brain wave changes and warn the person or a family member, it would greatly improve quality of life for many. For example, patients who are prone to harmful falls could be placed in a safe position. Early warning also may offer new types of treatment to stop seizures: electrical stimulation of the brain or vagus nerve could be triggered the seizure, or medications could be released "on demand" through a device implanted in the brain.

Supporting Epilepsy Research

Epilepsy research is underfunded. Although more than 750,000 Americans have uncontrolled epilepsy, research funding is relatively scarce and philanthropic support limited. The largest support comes from government grants, but more is badly needed. Individuals and small groups can help by writing to government representatives and strongly encouraging their support of epilepsy research. Several organizations actively support epilepsy research.

The Epilepsy Therapy Project (ETP) is dedicated to advancing new therapies for people with epilepsy. The ETP supports translational research grants to investigators in academic settings and industry who are pursuing projects that may lead to new therapeutic options or diagnostic techniques. This translational grant program is supported in collaboration with the Epilepsy Foundation and Finding a Cure for Epilepsy and Seizures (FACES). The ETP also makes direct investments in small companies that develop products to improve the lives of people with epilepsy. Together with FACES, the ETP also supports the Epilepsy Study Consortium (www.epilepsyconsortium.org), a group of scientific investigators from academic medical research centers dedicated to accelerating the development of new therapies in epilepsy. The organization's goals include building a partnership between academia, industry, and regulatory agencies and optimizing clinical trial methods to responsibly speed new treatments to patients.

The Epilepsy Foundation provides grants to epilepsy researchers in the early stages of their careers. Fellowship grants are available in several areas to promote epilepsy research.

FACES (www.med.nyu.edu/faces) is a non-profit affiliated with the NYU Epilepsy Center whose mission is to improve the quality of life for all people affected by epilepsy through research, clinical programs, education and awareness, and community-building events. Most research efforts are focused at NYU, although FACES also partners with the ETP and supports multicenter collaborative research ventures.

Citizens United for Epilepsy Research (CURE) is focused on supporting research and other initiatives toward a cure for epilepsy. CURE funds seed grants to young and established investigators to explore new areas and collect the data necessary to apply for further funding by the NIH.

The Partnership for Pediatric Epilepsy Research is a consortium formed by several organizations and individuals to promote innovative research into pediatric epilepsy, its causes, and potential avenues for new treatments and cures. Parents Against Childhood Epilepsy (PACE) supports research and educational programs to improve the lives of children with epilepsy.

Regional comprehensive epilepsy centers often conduct research studies. Support of these centers can be directed toward specific programs such as treatment of children with epilepsy or basic science research studies on epilepsy.

Future Advances in Understanding Epilepsy

The past few decades have shed new light on understanding the causes and mechanisms underlying seizures and epilepsy. Yet for the 30% of people whose seizures remain uncontrolled, advances in therapy have been painfully slow. The overall burden of refractory epilepsy remains very high. Most of the new AEDs are safer rather than more effective, although some provide seizure control where older AEDs did not.

Perhaps the greatest obstacle to finding a cure for epilepsy is the fragmented nature of medical research. Some of human being's greatest achievements, such as walking on the moon, were the result of very focused and intensive resources aimed at a specific goal. To cure epilepsy, we will need to bring our resources together and concentrate our efforts.

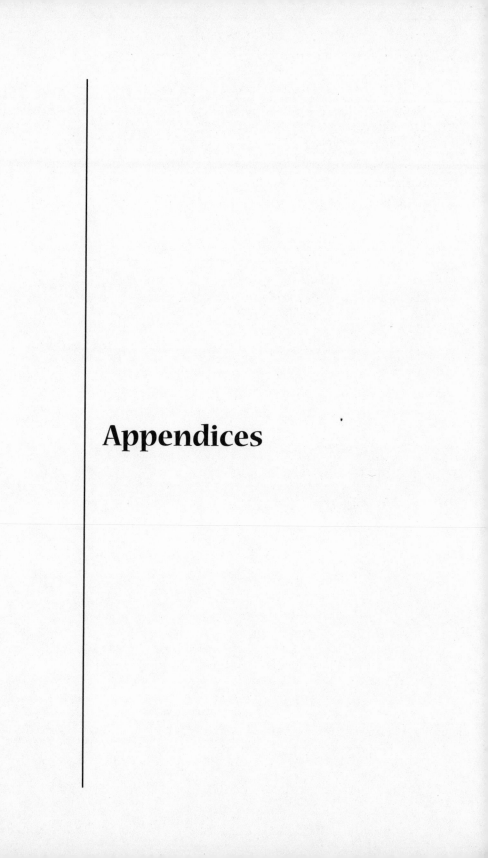

Appendices

A | The Brain and Epilepsy

T he human brain controls life support functions such as breathing and temperature regulation, survival behaviors such as eating and drinking, and sleep-wake cycles, emotions, sensations, movements, and intellect. Our *cerebral cortex* differs most from other animals' brains. The cortex forms the large outer surface of the brain, with numerous folds that increase the surface area (Fig. A1.1).

Anatomy of the Brain

The Cerebrum

The upper brain, or *cerebrum*, is composed of white matter and gray matter (Fig. A1.2). The gray matter forms the cerebral cortex and consists largely of nerve cells (*neurons*) and supportive cells (*glial cells*). The nerve cells work like computer chips, analyzing and processing information and then sending signals through the nerve fibers. The white matter lies beneath the cerebral cortex and is composed of nerve fibers. The nerve fibers act like telephone wires, connecting different areas of the brain, spinal cord, muscles, and glands.

The *cerebrum* is divided into left and right halves, called cerebral hemispheres. These are connected by a large white fiber bundle called the *corpus callosum* (see Fig. A1.2). Each cerebral hemisphere contains

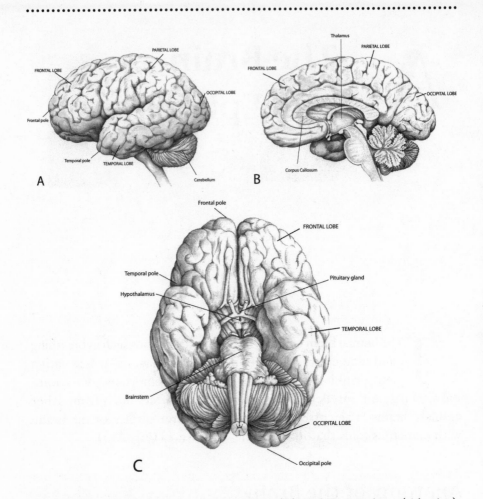

FIGURE A1.1: Three views of the brain. **(A)** Left hemisphere (*side view*). **(B)** Right hemisphere (*side view*). **(C)** Lower surface (*bottom view*).

four lobes: frontal, parietal, occipital, and temporal. Each lobe contains many different areas that have different functions. For example, in almost all right-handed persons, the area that controls speech lies in the left frontal lobe and the area that controls understanding of spoken and written language lies in the left temporal lobe. Brain functions are carried out by networks of related areas. If one area is injured, other related areas can often compensate. For example, the ability to focus our attention involves multiple cortical areas. Problems in certain critical areas of this "attention network" can severely disrupt the ability to stay focused. But disruption or damage in other, less critical areas

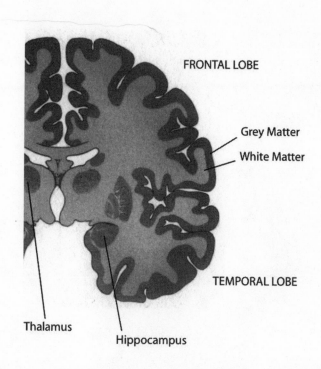

FIGURE A1.2: Cross section of the brain showing the gray matter and the white matter.

of the network will cause only a mild and temporary disorder. In contrast, some areas, such as those that control fine hand movements, are localized in only one area, and destruction of that area causes permanent impairments. The left half of the brain controls the right side of the body, and vice versa (Fig. A1.3). For example, a left cerebral stroke can cause weakness of the right arm and leg.

The outer regions of the cerebral cortex contain neocortex, including the sensory, motor, and cognitive ("thinking") areas. The deep, central portions of the frontal and temporal lobes contain the limbic cortex, which controls emotions and memory (Fig. A1.4C). Seizures can arise from limbic cortex or neocortex. The functions of the different parts of the brain are summarized in Figure A1.4.

Injury or disordered function of the cerebral cortex can cause seizures. If seizures arise from a specific area of the brain, then the initial symptoms of the seizure often reflect the functions of that

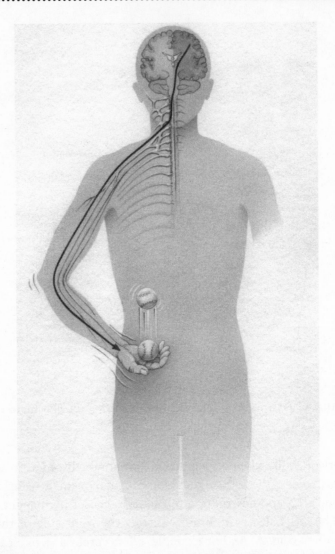

FIGURE A1.3: Nerve impulses originating from the left side of the brain control movements on the right side of the body and vice versa.

area. For example, if a seizure starts from the area of the right hemi-sphere that controls movements in the left thumb, then the seizure may begin with jerking movements of the left thumb or hand (Fig. A1.3). The motor cortex of each hemisphere is organized so that groups of muscles are controlled by specific areas. The lowest part controls the vocal cords and mouth, the middle part controls the hand and arm,

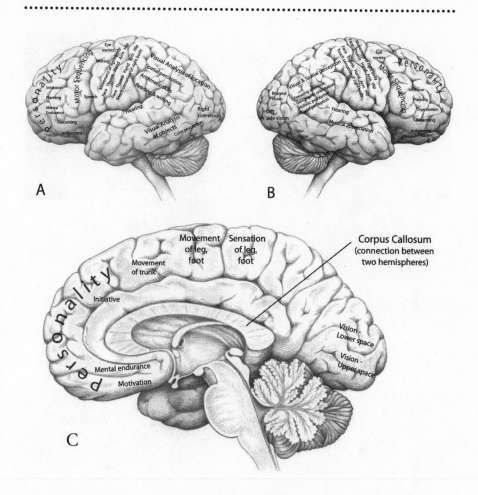

FIGURE A1.4: Areas of the human brain responsible for specific functions. **(A)** Left hemisphere (*side view*). **(B)** Right hemisphere (*side view*). **(C)** Inner surface (*cross-sectional view*). The areas in the frontal lobe and the side views of the parietal lobe are not as precisely distributed as the drawings indicate, and the areas overlap in their control of some functions.

and the upper part controls the leg on the opposite side of the body (Fig. A1.5).

The Brainstem and Spinal Cord

The lower part of the brain contains the *brainstem*, which controls sleep–wake cycles, breathing, and heartbeat. The upper part of the

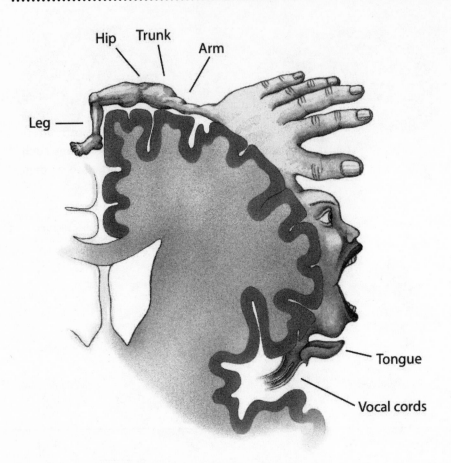

FIGURE A1.5: Drawing showing the parts of the body whose movements are controlled by various areas of the motor cortex in the right hemisphere.

brainstem contains the thalamus and hypothalamus (see Fig. A1.1B and C). The spinal cord begins as a continuation of the lower part of the brainstem.

The Thalamus

The thalamus processes sensory information, relaying information about bodily sensations to the cerebral cortex. It is also important in pain perception and in regulating the level of wakefulness (consciousness). The thalamus plays an important role in generalized epilepsies.

The Hypothalamus

The hypothalamus regulates endocrine (hormone) functions through its control over the pituitary gland. The hormones released by the pituitary gland control the activity of other endocrine glands, such as the ovaries, testicles, thyroid, and adrenal glands. The limbic areas of the temporal lobes influence the hypothalamus, which in turn alters pituitary gland functions. This explains why hormonal functions such as regulation of the menstrual cycle can be disrupted in some women with epilepsy.

The Lower Brainstem

The lower brainstem controls movement and sensation of the face, eye movements, taste, heartbeat, breathing, and other bodily functions.

The Cerebellum

The *cerebellum*, located behind the brainstem, helps coordinate and "automatize" complex movements.

The Spinal Cord

The spinal cord receives and sends information to the body about senses and movement.

The Central and Peripheral Nervous Systems

Together, the brain and spinal cord are called the central nervous system. The nerves in the face, arms, and legs make up the *peripheral nervous system.*

Nerve Cells of the Brain

Nerve cells (*neurons*) are the building blocks of the brain. There are approximately 35 billion nerve cells in the brain and spinal cord. Nerve cells are usually composed of three parts: the cell body, axon, and dendrites (Fig. A1.6). The cell body (*soma*) contains the enzymes and chemicals that regulate the cell's metabolism and genetic information. The *axon* is the long portion of a nerve cell that resembles a wire. Axons

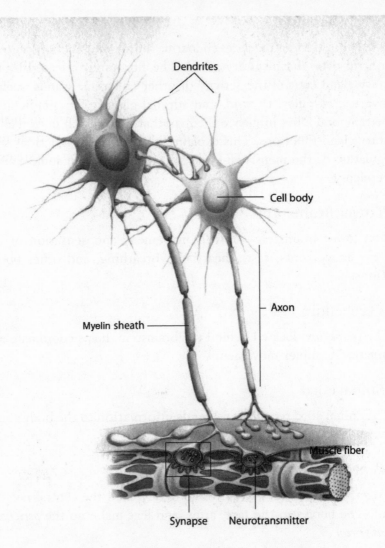

FIGURE A1.6: A neuron (nerve cell).

are the "transmitting" parts of the nerve fibers. Most axons are surrounded by myelin, a fatty covering, which insulates them like plastic around telephone wires—preventing "cross-talk."

Axons carry chemical messengers (neurotransmitters) from the cell body to the end of the axon, where they are released to influence other nerve cells. The space between the end of the axon and either a muscle or the dendrite of another neuron is the *synapse*. Dendrites are the neurons' "antennas." The neurotransmitters released from the axon travel across the synapse to interact with receptors on the muscle or dendrite.

Most nerve cells have thousands of synapses on their dendrites, with specific receptors for the different neurotransmitters to fit, like a key in a lock. A specific key is needed for a specific lock—there are no "master keys." Neurotransmitters may increase (excite) or decrease (inhibit) the cell's activity and thereby change the electrical activity and chemical composition of the cell. Thus, both electrical and chemical systems are critical for nerve cell functions and to transmit information.

Neurotransmitters

Neurotransmitters are the chemical messengers that work at the synapse. There are many kinds of neurotransmitters, but each individual nerve cell produces only one major type. Some of the neurotransmitters are carried a long distance within the nervous system. Others are produced by and released onto cells that are close to each other. Changes in certain neurotransmitter levels can make seizures more or less likely to occur.

Some neurotransmitters are *excitatory*—they stimulate or increase brain electrical activity and cause nerve cells to fire. Others are *inhibitory*—they shut off or decrease brain electrical activity and cause nerve cells to stop firing. Simplistically, epilepsy can be considered an imbalance between neurotransmitters that cause nerve cells to fire and those that cause them to stop firing. Either a deficiency of inhibitory neurotransmitters such as GABA or an excess of excitatory neurotransmitters such as glutamate increases the likelihood that a seizure will occur. Some AEDs target the increase of the inhibitory systems or the decrease of excitatory systems.

B | Antiepileptic Drugs

Generic name	Brand name	Indications
Acetazolamide (ah-seet-ah-**zole**-ah-myd)	Diamox (**dye**-ah-mox)	Myoclonic seizures Catamenial seizures
Adrenocortico-tropic hormone (ACTH)	Cortrosyn (**cor**-tro-sin)	Infantile spasms
Carbamazepine (kar-bah-**maz**-ah-peen)	Tegretol (**teh**-greh-tol) Carbatrol (car-bah-trol)	Partial seizures, tonic-clonic seizures
Clonazepam (kloh-**na**-zeh-pam)	Klonopin (**klah**-ni-pin)	Myoclonic seizures, absence seizures
Clorazepate (klor-**a**-zeh-pate)	Tranxene (**tran**-zeen)	Absence seizures, partial seizures
Diazepam (dye-**ah**-zah-pam)	Valium (oral) Diastat (rectal) (**dye**-ah-stat)	Seizure clusters, status epilepticus
Ethosuximide (eth-o-**sux**-i-mide)	Zarontin (za-**ron**-tin)	Absence seizures
Felbamate (**fel**-bah-mate)	Felbatol (**fel**-bah-tol)	Partial seizures, tonic-clonic seizures, atonic seizures, tonic seizures

(Continued)

Generic name	Brand name	Indications
Gabapentin (**gab**-ah-pen-tin)	Neurontin (nur-**on**-tin)	Partial seizures
Lamotrigine (lah-**mo**-tri-jeen)	Lamictal (lah-**mi**-ktal)	Partial seizures, tonic-clonic seizures, absence seizures
Leviteracetam	Keppra	Partial seizures, myoclonic seizures, tonic-clonic seizures
Lorazepam (lor-a-zeh-pam)	Ativan (**ah**-ti-van)	Status epilepticus, seizure clusters
Mephobarbital (meh-fo-**bar**-bi-tal)	Mebaral (**meh**-bah-ral)	Partial seizures, tonic-clonic seizures, myoclonic seizures
Oxcarbazepine (ox-car-**bah**-zeh-peen)	Trileptal (try-**lep**-tal)	Partial seizures, tonic-clonic seizures
Phenobarbital (fee-no-**bar**-bi-tal)	Luminal (and others) (**lu**-mih-nall)	Partial seizures, tonic-clonic seizures, myoclonic seizures
Phenytoin (**fen**-i-toe-in)	Dilantin (dye-**lan**-tin)	Partial seizures, tonic-clonic seizures
Pregabalin (pre-**gah**-bah-lin)	Lyrica (**leer**-i-cah)	Partial seizures
Prednisone (**pred**-nih-sone)	—	Infantile spasms
Primidone (**pri**-mi-done)	Mysoline (**my**-soh-leen)	Partial seizures, tonic-clonic seizures, myoclonic seizures
Tiagabine (ti-**ah**-gah-been)	Gabitril (**gab**-ih-tril)	Partial seizures, tonic-clonic seizures
Topiramate (toh-**peer**-ah-mate)	Topamax (**toh**-pah-maks)	Partial seizures, tonic-clonic seizures; infantile spasms, myoclonic seizures
Valproate (valproic acid; divalproex sodium)	Depakene (**deh**-pah-keen) Depakote (**deh**-pah-kote)	Absence seizures, tonic-clonic seizures, myoclonic seizures, partial seizures
Zonisamide (zoh-**nih**-sah-mide)	Zonegran (**zon**-ah-gran)	Partial seizures, tonic-clonic seizures, myoclonic seizures

C | Drug Interactions

Effects of Frequently Used Antiepileptic Drugs

AED	AED levels affects	Other interactions
Acetazolamide	*Increases* Carbamazepine Phenobarbital Phenytoin in children *Decreases* Primidone	May enhance bone loss when used with enzyme-inducing AEDs
Carbamazepine	*Decreases* Clobazam Clonazepam Diazepam Ethosuximide Felbamate Lamotrigine Phenobarbital Primidone Tiagabine Topirimate Valproate Zonisamide *Variable effect on* Phenytoin	Can potentiate neurotoxicity in combination with lamotrigine Additive cardiotoxicity with other Na-channel blockers, potential cardiotoxicity with calcium channel and beta-blockers *Decreases* OCPs, theophylline, coumadin

(Continued)

Effects of Frequently Used Antiepileptic Drugs (Continued)

AED	AED levels affects	Other interactions
Clonazepam		Benzodiazepines increase effects of other CNS depressants
Clorazepate	None	
Diazepam	*Decreases* Phenobabrital *Variable effect on* Phenytoin	Potentiates narcotic analgesics, barbiturates, phenothiazines, ethanol, antihistamines, MAO inhibitors, sedative-hypnotics, cyclic antidepressants
Ethosuximide	*Decreases* Valproate	Some interaction with fosphenytoin, phenobarbital, phenytoin
Felbamate	*Increases* Valproate, Phenobarbital Phenytoin *Decreases* Carbamazepine (but *increases* its meta-bolite CBZ-E, often causing side effects)	*Increases* Warfarin *Decreases* Effectiveness of oral contraceptives Felbamate and phenytoin have been reported to cause toxicity in two cases
Gabapentin	*Increases* Phenytoin (when taken with carbamazepine and clobazam)	
Lamotrigine	*Decreases* Valproate	Valproate with lamotrigine *increases* the risk of allergic rash and tremor Carbamazepine and lamotrigine can cause neurotoxicity
Levetiracetam	None	
Oxcarbazepine	*Decreases* Lamotrigine	*Decreases* Levels of oral contraceptives

(Continued)

Effects of Frequently Used Antiepileptic Drugs *(Continued)*

AED	AED levels affects	Other interactions
	Increases Phenobarbital Phenytoin	
Phenobarbital	*Decreases* Carbamazepine Clonazepam Ethosuximide Lamotrigine Oxcarbazepine metabolite Tiagabine Topirimate Valproate Zonisimide *Variable effect on* Phenytoin	*Decreases* Theophylline, coumarin, anticoagulants, steroids (including oral contraceptives), digoxin, cyclosporine, vitamin K, and tricyclic antidepressants, paroxetine (an SSRI)
Phenytoin	*Decreases* Carbamazepine Clobazam Clonazepam Ethosximide Felbamate Lamotrigine Oxcarbazepine Primidone Tiagabine Topirimate Tiagabine Valproate Zonisamide *Variable effect on* Diazepam, Phenobarbital	*Decreases* Amiodarone, estrogens, rifampin, Vitamin D, doxycycline, warfarin *Decreases* Effectiveness of oral contraceptives IV form with IV dopamine—severe hypotension, possibly cardiac arrest
Primidone	*Decreases* Carbamazepine Ethosuximide	Primidone is metabolized to phenobarbital, so has similar effects

(Continued)

Effects of Frequently Used Antiepileptic Drugs *(Continued)*

AED	AED levels affects	Other interactions
	Oxcarbazepine metabolite Lamotrigine Topiramate Tiagabine Valproate Zonisamide *Variable effect on* Phenytoin	*Decreases* Theophylline, coumarin anticoagulants, steroids (including oral contraceptives), digoxin, cyclosporine, vitamin K, and tricyclic antidepressants, paroxetine (an SSRI)
Tiagabine		
Topiramate	*Increases* Phenytoin *Decreases* Valproate	*Decreases* Extradiol , ethinyl estradiol in contraceptives, digoxin
Valproate	*Increases* Diazepam Lamotrigine Phenobarbital (including phenobarbital derived from primidone) Ethosuximide Carbamazepine *Decreases* Topirimate *Increases* Free fraction of phenytoin	Valproate with lamotrigine *increases* the risk of allergic rash and tremor
Vigabatrin	None	
Zonisamide		Concomitant administration of carbonic anhydrase inhibitors such as acetazolamide or topiramate may increase potential for renal stone formation

Effects of Other Medications on Seizure Medicines

Other medication	Seizure medicine affected
Acetaminophen	⇓ Lamotrigine
Aminophylline	⇓ Phenytoin
Amiodarone	⇓ Phenytoin
Amitryptiline	⇑ Carbamazepine
Cimetidine	⇑ Carbamazepine ⇑ Clobazam ⇑ Clonazepam ⇑ Clorazepate ⇑ Diazepam ⇑ Gabapentin by very little ⇑ Phenytoin
Ciprofloxacin	⇑ Diazepam ⇓ Phenytoin
Cisplatin	⇓ Carbamazepine
Clarithromycin	⇑ Carbamazepine ⇑ Clonazepam ⇑ Diazepam
Cloramphenicol	⇑ Carbatrol
Danazol	⇑ Carbamazepine
Desipramine	⇑ Carbamazepine
Diltiazem	⇑ Carbamazepine ⇑ Clonazepam ⇑ Diazepam +/- ⇑ Phenytoin
Disulfiram	⇑ Diazepam ⇑ Phenytoin
Doxepin	⇑ Carbamazepine

(Continued)

Effects of Other Medications on Seizure Medicines *(Continued)*

Other medication	Seizure medicine affected
Doxycycline	⇓ Carbamazepine
Erythromycin	⇑ Carbamazepine ⇑ Clonazepam ⇑ Diazepam
Ethanol	⇑ Diazepam
Fluconazole	⇑ Clonazepam ⇑ Clorazepate (when fluconazole is stopped) ⇑ Diazepam ⇑ Phenytoin
Fluoxetine	⇑ Carbamazepine ⇑ Phenytoin ⇑ Valproate
Fluvoxamine	⇑ Carbamazepine ⇑ Diazepam
Flurithromycin	⇑ Carbamazepine
Haloperidol	⇑ Carbamazepine +/- ⇓ Valproate
Isoniazid (INH)	⇑ Carbamazepine ⇑ Diazepam ⇑ Ethosuximide ⇑ Phenobarbital ⇑ Phenytoin ⇑ Primidone +/- ⇑ Valproate
Itraconazole	⇑ Diazepam ⇑ Phenytoin
Ketoconazole	⇑ Carbamazepine ⇑ Clonazepam ⇑ Diazepam

(Continued)

Effects of Other Medications on Seizure Medicines *(Continued)*

Other medication	Seizure medicine affected
Levodopa	⇑ Diazepam
Methotrexate	⇓ Phenytoin
Metronidazole	⇑ Carbamazepine ⇑ Diazepam ⇑ Phenytoin
Metropolol	⇑ Diazepam
Miconazole + flucytosine	⇑ Phenytoin
Nefazadone	⇑ Carbamazepine
Nicotinamide	⇑ Carbamazepine ⇑ Primidone
Nortryptiline	⇑ Carbamazepine
Omeprazole	⇑ Diazepam +/- ⇑ Phenytoin
Panipenem-betamipron	⇓ Valproate
Phenylbutazone	⇑ Free Phenytoin ⇓ Phenobarbital
Propoxyphene	⇑ Phenytoin +/- ⇑ Phenobarbital with high dosage ⇑ Carbamazepine
Pyridoxine	⇓ Phenobarbital (from primidone metabolism)
Quinine	⇑ Phenobarbital
Ranitidine	+/- ⇑ Phenytoin,
Rifabutin	⇓ Clonazepam ⇓ Diazepam

(Continued)

Effects of Other Medications on Seizure Medicines *(Continued)*

Other medication	Seizure medicine affected
Rifampin	⇊ Clonazepam ⇊ Clorazepate ⇊ Diazepam ⇊ Ethosuximide ⇊ Lamotrigine ⇊ Phenobarbital (from primidone metabolism) ⇊ Phenytoin
Risperidone	May react with valproate to cause swelling
Ritonavir	⇈ Clonazepam
Sertraline	⇈ Lamotrigine ⇈ Phenytoin
Sucralfate	⇊ Phenytoin
Sulfa drugs	⇊ Phenytoin
Theophylline	⇊ Carbamazepine
Ticlopidine	⇈ Carbamazepine ⇈ Phenytoin
Troleandomycin	⇈ Carbamazepine
Trimethoprim	⇈ Phenytoin
Troleandomycin	⇈ Carbamazepine
Verapamil	⇈ Carbamazepine ⇈ Clonazepam ⇈ Diazepam
Viloxazine	⇈ Carbamazepine ⇈ Phenytoin
Vinblastine	⇊ Phenytoin

KEY: ⇊ Level of seizure medicine in the blood is decreased.
⇈ Level of seizure medicine in the blood is increased.
+/- Variable or mild effect not seen in all patients; rarely affects how patients feel or their condition.

Selected Over-the-Counter Drugs and Foods That Can Affect Seizure Control or Drug Side Effects

Drug/Food	Effect	Common products*
Acetaminophen	Slight decrease level of lamotrigine	Alka-Seltzer Drixoral Excedrin Midol Robitussin Sudafed TheraFlu Tylenol
Aspirin or other salicylates†	Slight decrease total level of phenytoin but slight increase free level May increase levels of valproate in the blood	Alka-Seltzer Anacin Bayer Aspirin Bufferin Excedrin
Diphenhydramine	Can lower seizure threshold (minimum conditions necessary to produce a seizure)	Alka-Seltzer PM Pain Reliever and Sleep Aid Benadryl Goody's PM Powder Nytol Sominex Tylenol PM
Grapefruit juice	*Increases* level of carbamazepine in the blood, causing side effects	
Phenylephrine	Potential to lower seizure threshold	Sudafed, Robitussin Tylenol Sinus, DayQuil
Pseudoephedrine	Potential to lower seizure threshold	Sudafed, Decofed Drixoral, Ridafed

*These are not all-inclusive lists. Refer to ingredient lists when determining whether a product may affect seizure control or contribute to side effects of drugs.

†Low to moderate doses of aspirin (less than 1500 mg/day) are generally very safe for people who take antiepileptic drugs. Higher doses should only be taken after discussion with a doctor, especially if phenytoin or valproate is used. Aspirin-free versions of some products listed are available.

D | Resources for People with Epilepsy

General

Epilepsy.com
Internet site for patients and families affected by epilepsy. Includes basic to much more advanced information and videos. Large online community section
www.epilepsy.com

The Epilepsy Foundation
General information and online community section
8301 Professional Place
Landover, MO 20785
(800) 332-1000
(301) 459-3700
www.epilepsyfoundation.org

Epilepsy Information Service
Medical Center Boulevard
Winston-Salem, NC 27157-1078
(800) 642-0500

Medicine-On-Time
10085 Red Run Boulevard, Suite 109
Owings Mills, MD 21117
(800) 722-8824 voice
(800) 386-8788 fax
www.medicine-on-time.com

National Epilepsy Library
The Epilepsy Foundation
4351 Garden City Drive
Landover, MD 20785
(800) EFA-4050

National Library of Medicine
Excellent site for abstracts of medical articles
8600 Rockville Pike
Bethesda, MD 20894
www.nlm.nih.gov
www.ncbi.nlm.nih.gov/PubMed

General—Child

Children's Defense Fund
25 E Street, NW
Washington, DC 20001
(202) 628-8787
www.childrensdefense.org/

The Council for Exceptional Children
1110 North Glebe Road, Suite 300
Arlington, VA 22201-5704
Toll-free:1-888-CEC-SPED
Local: (703) 620-3660
www.cec.sped.org

Danmar Products, Inc. (Custom head protection)
221 Jackson Industrial Drive
Ann Arbor, MI 48103

(800) 783-1998
www.danmarproducts.com

Kids on the Block, Inc. (Educational puppet programs)
9385-C Gerwig Lane
Columbia, MD 21046-1583
Call: (800) 368-KIDS (5437)
or (410) 290-9095
FAX: (410) 290-9358
www.kotb.com

The National Information Center for Children and Youth with Disabilities
P.O. Box 1492
Washington, DC 20013-1492
(800) 695-0285 (Voice/TTY)
or (202) 884-8200 (Voice/TTY)
www.nichcy.org

Related Neurologic and Metabolic Disorders

(Alphabetical, by Disease)

National Angelman Syndrome Foundation
414 Plaza Drive, Suite 209
Westmont, IL 60559
(800) 432-6435
or (630) 734-9267
www.angelman.org
www.asclepius.com/angel/asfinfo.html (Related information site)

Autism Society of America
7910 Woodmont Avenue, Suite 300
Bethesda, MD 20814-3067
(301) 657-0881 or (800) 3AUTISM
www.autism-society.org/

Autism-PDD Resources Network
www.autism-pdd.net/

National Brain Tumor Foundation
www.braintumor.org

Cerebral Cavernous Malformations
Website of Angioma Alliance
www.angiomaalliance.org

United Cerebral Palsy
1660 L Street, NW, Suite 700
Washington, DC 20036
www.ucpa.org

The National Fragile X Foundation
P.O. Box 190488
San Francisco, CA 94119
(800) 688-8765
(510) 763-6030
www.nfxf.org

Learning Disabilities Association of America, Inc.
4156 Library Road
Pittsburgh, PA 15234
 (412) 341-1515
(412) 344-0224 (Fax)
www.ldanatl.org

National Alliance for the Mentally Ill (NAMI)
Colonial Place Three
2107 Wilson Blvd., Suite 300
Arlington, VA 22201-3042
NAMI HelpLine: 1-800-950-NAMI (6264)
Main Office: (703)524-7600
Fax: (703)524-9094
TDD: (703)516-7227
www.nami.org/

Mental Retardation–Association for Retarded Citizens (The Arc)
2501 Avenue J
Arlington, TX 76011

(871) 640-0204
www.thearc.org

United Mitochondrial Disease Foundation
P.O. Box 1151
Monroeville, PA 15146-1151
(412) 793-8077
www.umdf.org

National Institute of Neurological Disorders and Stroke
NIH Neurological Institute
P.O. Box 5801
Bethesda, MD 20824
Phone: (800) 352-9424
www.ninds.nih.gov

Neurofibromatosis—The Children's Tumor Foundation
Ending Neurofibromatosis Through Research
www.ctf.org

The Sturge–Weber Foundation
P.O. Box 418
Mount Freedom, NJ 07970
(800) 627-5482
or (973) 895-4445
www.sturge-weber.com/

Tuberous Sclerosis Alliance
801 Roeder Road, Suite 750
Silver Spring, MD 20910
(800) 225-6872
or (301) 562-9890
www.tsalliance.org
www.stsn.nl/tsi/tsi.htm (International site)

Williams Syndrome Association
P.O. Box 297
Clawson, MI 48017-0297
(248) 541-3630
www.williams-syndrome.org/welcome.html

Career and Rehabilitation

Americans with Disability Act
Department of Justice
P.O. Box 66118
Washington, DC 20035
(202) 514-0301
www.usdoj.gov/crt/ada/adahom1.htm

Access America for People with Disabilities
Website established by Presidential Task Force on Employment of Adults
with Disabilities, with extensive information and links to government
services.
www.disAbility.gov

DisabilityResources.org
www.disabilityresources.org/EMPLOYMENT.html
(Information on employment discrimination)
www.disabilityresources.org/DRMreg.html
(State listing of agencies for people with disabilities)

The Job Accommodation Network (JAN)
918 Chestnut Ridge Road, Suite 1
West Virginia University, P.O. Box 6080
Morgantown, WV 26506
(800) 526-7234
www.jan.wvu.edu

National Organization on Disability
910 Sixteenth Street, NW, Suite 600
Washington, DC 20006
(202) 293-5960 or (202) 293-5968 TTY
www.nod.org

National Rehabilitation Information Center (NARIC)
8455 Colesville Road, Suite 935
Silver Spring, MD 20910
(800) 346-2742
or (301) 495-5626 TTY
www.cais.com/naric

Rehabilitation Services Administration (RSA)

Office of Special Education and Rehabilitation Service (OSERS)
U.S. Department of Education
Switzer Building
330 C Street, SW
Washington, DC 20202
(202) 205-5465 (Voice or TTY)
www.ed.gov/offices/OSERS/RSA/rsa.html

Social Security Administration

(800) 772-1213 or (800) 325-0778 TTY
www.ssa.gov/regions/regional.html (Regional offices)
www.ssa.gov/disability/ (Social Security Disability Insurance [SSDI])
www.ssa.gov/notices/supplemental-security-income/ (Supplemental
Security Income [SSI])

The U.S. Equal Employment Opportunity Commission (EEOC)

1801 L Street, N.W.
Washington, D.C. 20507
(202) 663-4900
(800) 669-4000 or (800) 669-6820 TTY
(To be connected to the nearest field office)
www.eeoc.gov/

Young Adult Institute (YAI) / National Institute for People with Disabilities

Central Office
460 West 34th Street
New York, NY 10001-2382
(212) 563-7474
www.YAI.org

Pharmacies—Mail-Order and Online

AARP Pharmacy Service from Retired Persons Services, Inc.

(800) 456-2277
www.aarppharmacy.com

Caligor Pharmacy (Specializing in foreign medications)
1226 Lexington Ave.
New York, NY 10028
(212) 369-6000

drugstore.com
(800) 378-4786
www.drugstore.com

Express Scripts
(800) 441-8976
https://www.express-scripts.com/prescriptions/prescriptions.htm

Neurologic and Metabolic Disorders

Autism
Autism Society of America
www.autism-society.org/

Cerebral Cavernous Malformations
The website of the Angioma Alliance, a group dedicated to providing education, networking and support opportunities, and research information for people with clusters of abnormal blood vessels in the brain or spine.
www.angiomaalliance.org

Cerebral Palsy
UCP (United Cerebral Palsy): Organization that works to advance the independence, productivity and full citizenship of people with cerebral palsy and other disabilities. Site offers information on local as well as national services.
www.ucp.org/index.cfm

Fragile X
The National Fragile X Foundation
www.nfxf.org/

Hypothalamic Hamartoma

Hypothalamic Hamartoma Support Group: Information and support site operated by families of children or adults with this rare disorder.
www.geocities.com/hhugs2001/index.htm

Learning Disabilities

Learning Disabilities Association of America
www.ldanatl.org/

Mental Illness

National Alliance for the Mentally Ill (NAMI): Support and advocacy organization working to improve the lives of people with severe mental illnesses.
www.nami.org/

Mental Retardation

The Arc of the United States: National organization of and for people with mental retardation and related developmental disabilities and their families.
www.thearc.org/

The Joseph P. Kennedy, Jr. Foundation

Services for those with mental retardation.
www.jpkf.org/

Mitochondrial Disease

United Mitochondrial Disease Foundation
www.umdf.org

Neurofibromatosis

The Children's Tumor Foundation:Ending Neurofibromatosis Through Research (formerly known as the National Neurofibromatosis Foundation).
www.ctf.org

Stroke and Other Disorders

National Institute of Neurological Disorders and Stroke
www.ninds.nih.gov

National Stroke Association
www.stroke.org

Sturge-Weber Syndrome
The Sturge-Weber Foundation promotes research and services for individuals with Sturge-Weber syndrome, Port Wine Stains, and Klippel-Trenauney syndrome.
www.sturge-weber.com/

Glossary

Absence seizure: A primary generalized epileptic seizure, usually lasting less than 20 seconds, characterized by a stare sometimes associated with blinking or brief automatic movements of the mouth or hands; formerly called *petit mal* seizure. Usually begin in childhood, usually easily controlled with medication, and are often outgrown. *See* Atypical absence seizure.

Accommodation (or Reasonable accommodation): Any change in the work environment or in the way things are customarily done that enables an individual with a disability to enjoy equal employment opportunities.

ADA: *See* Americans with Disabilities Act.

ADD: *See* Attention deficit disorder.

ADHD: Attention deficit/hyperactivity disorder.

Adjunct: Something added to another thing in a subordinate position or use; for example, an adjunct drug is one used in addition to another drug, not alone (*add-on therapy*).

Adverse effects: The undesirable or unfavorable effects of something; side effects.

AED: Antiepileptic drug.

Ambulatory EEG monitoring: Recording of the EEG for a prolonged period in an outpatient.

Americans with Disabilities Act: A law that makes discrimination against people with disabilities illegal; the act applies to employment and access to public places.

Antiepileptic drug: A medication used to control both convulsive and nonconvulsive seizures.

Atonic seizure: An epileptic seizure characterized by sudden loss of muscle tone; may cause head drop, objects to fall from the hands, or falling.

Attention deficit disorder (ADD): An impairment in the ability to focus or maintain attention.

Atypical absence seizure: A staring spell characterized by partial impairment of consciousness; often occurs in children with the Lennox-Gastaut syndrome.

Aura: A warning before a seizure; a simple partial seizure occurring within seconds or minutes before a complex partial or secondarily generalized tonic-clonic seizure, or it may occur alone; also a warning before a migraine headache or a primary generalized seizure.

Autoinduction (of metabolism): A process in which continued administration of a drug leads to an increase in the rate at which the drug is metabolized (e.g., carbamazepine).

Automatism: Automatic, involuntary movement during a seizure; may involve mouth, hand, leg, or body movements; consciousness is usually impaired; occurs during complex partial and absence seizures and after tonic-clonic seizures.

Autonomic: Pertaining to the autonomic nervous system, which controls bodily functions that are not under conscious control (for example, heartbeat, breathing, sweating).

Autosomal dominant: A mode of inheritance in which a gene is passed on by either parent; in most cases, the child has a 50% chance of inheriting the gene; the *expression* of the gene (that is, the development of the physical trait or the disorder) can vary among different individuals with the same gene.

Autosomal recessive: A mode of inheritance in which an individual has two copies of a gene that requires both copies for *expression* of the trait. Both parents must be *carriers* (only one copy of the gene but do not have the physical trait) or have the trait (two copies of the gene).

Axon: The part of the nerve cell (neuron) that communicates with other cells, similar to a telephone wire; the axon is often covered with myelin, an insulating fatty layer.

Benign: Favorable for recovery.

Benign rolandic epilepsy: An epilepsy syndrome of childhood characterized by partial seizures occurring at night and often involving the face and tongue; characteristic EEG pattern, easily controlled with medications but may not require treatment; outgrown by age 16 years.

Blood drug level: The concentration, or amount, of circulating drug in the bloodstream, measured in micrograms (µg) or nanograms (ng) per milliliter (mL). The *free level* is the amount that is "free" (unbound); the *total level* is the amount that is both bound and unbound to the blood protein; the drug that is free (unbound) is the portion that reaches the brain.

Brand-name drug: Medication manufactured by a major pharmaceutical company; the drugs are often expensive but tend to be more uniform than generics.

Breath-holding spells: Harmless episodes in children in which intense emotional upset is followed by interruption of breathing and sometimes loss of consciousness and jerking.

Catamenial: Referring to the menses or to menstruation; catamenial epilepsy is a tendency for seizures at certain times of the menstrual cycle.

Cerebral hemisphere: One side of the cerebrum (upper brain). Each hemisphere contains four lobes: frontal, parietal, occipital, and temporal.

Cerebral palsy: A condition with combinations of impaired muscle tone and strength, coordination, and intelligence.

Clonic seizure: An epileptic seizure characterized by jerking movements and involving muscles on both sides.

Cognitive: Pertaining to the mental processes of perceiving, thinking, and remembering; i.e., intellectual functions.

Complex partial seizure: An epileptic seizure that involves part of the brain and impairs consciousness; often preceded by a simple partial seizure (aura or warning) and accompanied by automatisms.

Computed tomography (CT): A scanning technique that uses x-rays and computers to create pictures of the inside of the body; not as sensitive as MRI.

Consciousness: State of awareness; if consciousness is preserved during a seizure, the person can respond and recall what occurred during the spell.

Controlled study: An experiment in which two groups are the same except that only one receives the drug, treatment, etc., being tested.

Convulsion: An older term for a tonic-clonic seizure.

Convulsive syncope: A fainting episode in which the brain does not receive enough blood, causing a seizure, but not an epileptic seizure.

Corpus callosotomy: Surgery that disconnects the cerebral hemispheres and reduces atonic and tonic-clonic seizures.

Cortical dysplasia: An abnormality in the development and organization of the cerebral cortex that can cause seizures and other neurologic disorders.

CT scan: *See* Computed tomography.

Daily dose: The daily amount of medication taken.

Deficit: A lack or deficiency of an essential quality or element; for example, arm weakness is a neurologic deficit.

Deja vu: Feeling as if one has lived through or experienced this moment before; may occur in people without any medical problems or as a simple partial seizure.

Development: The process of physical and mental growth that begins in infancy; any interruption of this process by a disease or disorder is called *developmental delay*.

Dose-related effects: Side effects that are more likely to occur at times of peak blood levels of a drug.

EEG: *See* Electrocencephalogram.

EEOC: Equal Employment Opportunity Commission.

EF: Epilepsy Foundation.

Electrode: A conductor through which electrical current enters or leaves. When used to record the electroencephalogarm, a small metal disc attached to a wire is usually used.

Electroencephalogram (EEG): A diagnostic test of brain electrical activity; helpful in diagnosing epilepsy.

Elimination: The removal of waste products from the body.

Encephalitis: A brain inflammation usually caused by a virus.

Epilepsia partialis continua: A continuous or prolonged partial seizure that causes muscle contractions; usually restricted to the face, arm, or leg.

Epilepsy: A disorder characterized by a tendency toward (two or more) seizures.

Epilepsy syndrome: A disorder defined by seizure type, age of onset, clinical and EEG findings, family history, response to therapy, and prognosis.

Epileptiform: Resembling epilepsy or its manifestations; often refers to EEG patterns.

Epileptogenic: Causing epilepsy.

Epileptologist: A neurologist with specialty training in epilepsy.

Equilibrium period: *See* Steady state.

ETP: Epilepsy Therapy Project.

Excitatory: Stimulating or increasing brain electrical activity; causing nerve cells to fire.

FACES: Finding a Cure for Epilepsy and Seizures.

Febrile seizure: A seizure associated with high fever in children aged 3 months to 6 years, usually a tonic-clonic seizure; usually benign.

Fit: An older term for a seizure, usually a tonic-clonic seizure.

Focal seizure: An older term for a partial seizure.

Focus: The center or region of the brain from which seizures begin; used in reference to partial seizures.

Generalized seizure: A seizure that involves both sides of the brain and causes tonic and clonic movements (primary or secondary generalized) or another type of primary generalized epilepsy (e.g., absence or atonic seizure).

Generic drug: A drug that is not sold under a brand name; often less expensive, but uniformity of amount of drug and methods of preparation may be less than the brand name.

Grand mal: An older term for a tonic-clonic seizure.

Half-life: The time required for the amount of a drug in the blood to decline to half of its original value, measured in hours.

Hemispherectomy: A surgical procedure to remove and/or disconnect a cerebral hemisphere (one side of the brain).

Hereditary: Traits that are passed through the genes.

Hydrocephalus: A condition associated with excess cerebrospinal fluid within the skull.

Hyperventilation: Increased rate and depth of breathing; may be done during the EEG to increase the chances of finding epileptiform or other abnormal activity.

Hypsarrhythmia: An abnormal EEG pattern of excessive slow activity and multiple areas of epileptiform activity; associated with infantile spasms.

Ictal: Referring to the period during a sudden attack, such as a seizure or stroke.

Idiopathic: Referring to a disorder of unknown cause.

Idiosyncratic: Pertaining to an abnormal susceptibility to some effect (e.g. of a drug) peculiar to the individual.

Incidence: The number of new cases of a disorder occurring in a population during a specified period.

Individuals with Disabilities Education Act (IDEA): U.S. law ensuring that handicapped children receive appropriate education at no cost and in the least restrictive environment.

Infantile spasm: A sudden jerk followed by stiffening; spasms usually begin between age 3 and 12 months and usually stop by age 2–4 years, although other seizure types often develop.

Inhibitory: Shutting off or decreasing brain electrical activity; causing nerve cells to stop firing.

Intensive monitoring: *See* Video-EEG monitoring.

Interictal: Referring to the period between seizures.

Intractable: Difficult to alleviate, remedy, or cure; for example, intractable seizures are difficult to control with AEDs.

Intravenous infusion: Administering a drug or other substance as part of a liquid solution injected directly into a vein.

Investigational drug: A drug available only for experimental purposes to test its safety and effectiveness.

JME: *See* Juvenile myoclonic epilepsy.

Juvenile myoclonic epilepsy (JME): A primary generalized epilepsy syndrome, usually beginning between ages 5 and 17 years, characterized by myoclonic (muscle-jerk) seizures and possibly also absence and tonic-clonic seizures.

Ketogenic diet: A high-fat, low-carbohydrate diet used to control seizures.

Kindling: A process in experimental animals in which intermittent electrical shocks cause a progressive tendency toward seizures.

Landau-Kleffner syndrome: A disorder of childhood characterized by the regression of language milestones in association with frequent epilepsy waves on the EEG.

Lennox-Gastaut syndrome: A disorder beginning in childhood, characterized by developmental delay or mental retardation, multiple seizure types that do not respond well to therapy, and slow spike-and-wave discharges on the EEG.

Magnetic resonance imaging (MRI): A scanning technique that creates pictures of the inside of the body and the brain; uses a strong magnet; more sensitive than CT.

Magnetic resonance spectroscopy (MRS): A scanning technique that examines the atoms hydrogen and phosphorus to measure chemical activity in small areas of brain.

Magnetoencephalography (MEG): Recording the brain's magnetic activity.

Mainstream: Regular (public, private, or parochial) school or classes.

Medical history: The account of a patient's disorder.

Meningitis: A bacterial infection of the membranes surrounding the brain; often diagnosed by a spinal tap (lumbar puncture).

Metabolism: The processes by which substances are produced or transformed (broken down) into energy or products.

Metabolite: Chemical product derived from breakdown (metabolism) of another chemical; may be biologically *active* or *inactive*.

Migraine: A headache characterized by throbbing head pain, often greater on one side; may be preceded by a warning (aura) and accompanied by nausea, vomiting, and sensitivity to light and sound.

Minor (motor) seizure: An older term for seizures that cause contraction of muscles but do not become tonic-clonic seizures.

Monotherapy: Treatment with a single medication.

Motor: Of or relating to movements of the muscles; of, pertaining to, or designating nerves carrying impulses to the muscles.

MRI: *See* Magnetic resonance imaging.

Muscle tone: The level of muscle contraction present during the resting state; with *increased tone* there is stiffness and rigidity; with *decreased tone* there is looseness of the limbs and trunk.

Myoclonic jerk: Brief muscle jerk; may involve muscles on one or both sides of the body; may be normal (for example, as one falls asleep) or caused by a seizure or other disorders.

Myoclonic seizure: A brief muscle jerk resulting from an abnormal discharge of brain electrical activity.

Narcolepsy: A condition characterized by sudden and uncontrollable attacks of sleep.

Neuron: A nerve cell.

Neurotransmitter: A chemical substance produced by nerve cells, causes chemical and electrical changes in adjacent cells.

Paroxysmal: Pertaining to a sudden outburst, such sudden symptoms or epileptiform activity on the EEG.

Partial complex seizure: Same as complex partial seizure.

Partial seizure: A seizure arising from part of the brain.

Peak blood level: The highest concentration of a drug in the bloodstream.

PET: *See* Positron emission tomography.

Petit mal: An older term for absence seizure.

Pharmacology: The study of drugs, including their effectiveness, side effects, metabolism, and interactions.

Photic stimulation: Shining, flashing (strobe) lights in the eyes (which may be closed) of a person; used during the EEG to detect photosensitive epilepsy.

Photosensitive epilepsy: A form of reflex epilepsy in which lights, especially flashing lights, can provoke seizures.

Positron emission tomography (PET): A diagnostic test that uses a very low dose of a radioactive compound to measure metabolic activity in the brain; areas of decreased metabolism correspond to the seizure focus.

Postictal: Referring to the period immediately after a seizure.

Predisposition: Tendency or inclination.

Premonitory: Serving as a warning.

Prevalence: The number of cases of a disorder present in a population at a specified time.

Primary drug: A drug that is well established for safely and effectively treating a particular disorder.

Prognosis: The outlook for a medical condition; the chances the condition will improve, remain unchanged, or worsen.

Progressive: Increasing in scope or severity over time.

Progressive myoclonic epilepsy: A rare group of epilepsies, often inherited characterized by myoclonic and other seizures and progressive neurologic impairment.

Psychic: Pertaining to intellectual or emotional (affective) functions.

Psychogenic (nonepileptic; pseudo) seizure: A behavioral episode that resembles an epileptic seizure but does not result from abnormal brain electrical activity; psychological in origin, but not resulting from conscious actions.

Psychomotor seizure: An older term for a complex partial seizure with automatism.

Rasmussen's syndrome: A disorder with frequent or continuous partial seizures and a progressive abnormality in the brain, possibly the result of a virus or autoimmune process.

Reflex epilepsy: Seizures precipitated by certain conditions or stimuli, such as flashing lights or loud sounds.

Refractory: A condition that does not respond easily to treatment.

Secondary drug: A drug whose efficacy and/or safety are not as good as a primary drug.

Seizure: A sudden, excessive discharge of nervous-system electrical activity that usually causes a change in behavior.

Seizure threshold: Minimal conditions necessary to produce a seizure.

Sensory: Pertaining to the senses (touch, vision, hearing, taste, smell).

Sharp wave: An EEG pattern indicating the potential for epilepsy; "benign" sharp waves are not associated with seizures.

Sibling: A brother or sister.

Simple partial seizure: An epileptic seizure that involves only part of the brain and does not impair consciousness.

Single-photon emission computed tomography (SPECT): A diagnostic test that uses a very low dose of a radioactive compound to measure blood flow in the brain.

Slowing: A term used for brain waves on the EEG that have a lower frequency than expected, can result from drowsiness or sleep, drugs, or brain injuries and occur during or after seizures.

Social Security Disability Income (SSDI): A federal assistance program for disabled people who have paid Social Security taxes or are dependents of people who have paid.

SPECT: *See* Single-photon emission computed tomography.

Spell: A period, bout, or episode of illness or indisposition.

Spike: An EEG pattern strongly correlated with seizures; "benign" spikes are not associated with seizures.

SSA: Social Security Administration.

SSDI: *See* Social Security Disability Income.

SSI: *See* Supplemental Security Income.

Status epilepticus: A prolonged seizure (usually defined as lasting longer than 5–10 minutes) or a series of repeated seizures; a continuous state of seizure activity.

Steady state: A state in which equilibrium has been achieved.

Sturge-Weber syndrome: A disorder of blood vessels affecting the skin of the face, eyes, and brain; brain involvement is associated with seizures.

Supplemental Security Income (SSI): A federal assistance program.

Symptomatic: A disorder with an identifiable cause; for example, head trauma can cause symptomatic epilepsy.

Synapse: The junction between one nerve cell and another nerve cell; the axon of one nerve cell releases a neurotransmitter, which diffuses across the synapse and causes changes in the membrane of the adjacent cell.

Syncope: Fainting.

Syndrome: A group of signs and symptoms that collectively define or characterize a disease or disorder; signs are objective findings such as weakness, and symptoms are subjective findings such as a feeling of fear.

Temporal lobe epilepsy: Partial epilepsy arising from the temporal lobe.

Temporal lobe seizure: A simple or complex partial seizure arising from the temporal lobe.

Therapeutic blood level: The amount of drug circulating in the bloodstream that brings about seizure control without troublesome side effects in most patients.

Threshold: The level at which an event or change occurs (*see* Seizure threshold).

Tic: Repeated involuntary contractions of muscles, such as rapid head jerks or eye blinks; nonepileptic.

Time to Peak Blood Level: The time drug is taken its highest concentration in the blood.

Todd's paralysis: Weakness after a seizure; originally used to describe muscle weakness on one side of the body, but now used to describe a variety of temporary problems after seizures such as blindness or loss of speech.

Tolerance: Decreased sensitivity to the effects of a substance such as a drug.

Tone: *See* Muscle tone.

Tonic seizure: An epileptic seizure that causes stiffening on both sides of the body, and electrical discharge involves all or most of the brain.

Tonic-clonic seizure: A convulsion; newer term for grand mal or major motor seizure; characterized by loss of consciousness, falling, stiffening, and jerking.

Trauma: An injury or wound caused by external force.

Tuberous sclerosis: A disease in which benign tumors affect the brain, eyes, skin, and internal organs; associated with mental retardation and seizures; may be inherited.

Vagus nerve stimulator (VNS): A pacemaker-like device, implanted in the upper chest, which stimulates a nerve in the left neck and can reduce seizure activity.

Video-EEG monitoring: A technique for recording the behavior and the EEG of a patient simultaneously; changes in behavior can be correlated with changes in the EEG.

West's syndrome: An epileptic syndrome characterized by infantile spasms, mental retardation, and an abnormal EEG pattern (hypsarrhythmia); begins before 1 year of age.

Index